Learning Victories

Conquering Dyslexic, Attention Deficit and Learning Challenges

Comments on *Learning Victories*

"*Learning Victories* is an excellent guide for therapists, teachers and parents. The exercises are wonderful and easy-to -use. It would be a great book for prospective teachers to read, in order to increase their sensitivity to learning difficulties that they will find in their students. Experienced teachers would benefit equally.

I was especially fascinated by the testimonials of Melody and Tim - I feel almost as if I know them by now. Melody's "Meadow Musing" is incredible! How rewarding it must be for you as a therapist. It is such a validation of your philosophy, your approach, your sensitivity, and your teaching. Your goal to share your vision, and create new believers and teachers, will result in many learning victories for many grateful people."

Principal and Educational Consultant

"*Learning Victories* is a great sequel to *You Don't Have to Be Dyslexic*. It is a valuable handbook for teachers, educational therapists, and parents, who are serious about working with children and adults who have learning inefficiencies. I have found Dr. Joan Smith's approach in using Edu-Therapeutics and diet modification to be very beneficial in remediating learning challenges for students and adults who have tried it."

Educator and Parent

Comments on *Edu-Therapeutics*

"*I have been working with students who have learning differences for two years. Before I attended the intensive Edu-Therapeutics training and became certified in this wonderful program, I had received some excellent training. I felt that I had some good methods of teaching kids reading and comprehension. However, I still felt frustrated and that something was missing.*

Since completing and implementing the training I received (and continue to receive) from Joan Smith and her staff, I feel that the missing pieces have fallen into place. My tutoring practice is now full, and I am confident that I am using powerful methods to help each of my students with his or her own particular needs. I feel deep gratitude and appreciation for Joan and her staff. Joan is so clearly committed to making a difference in this world, and she continues to be a source of support, encouragement and inspiration for me in my work with kids."

Certified Dyslexia Remediation Specialist

"*After twenty-five years as a special education teacher, I can return to the idealism of my early years with a tool bag that is practical and complete. It has rekindled by career... I even look younger !!!*"

Resource Specialist and Certified D.R.S.

Learning Victories

Resolving Dyslexic, Attention Deficit and Learning Challenges

Dr. Joan Smith

Learning Time Products, Inc.
Sacramento, California
1998

DEDICATION

It is my joy and privilege to be surrounded with believers. It is these individuals who nourish and stoke my energy. They bring me the questions and ignite my curiosity to find the answers. I thank them for their trust.

This books is dedicated to them

Cathy, Sandra, Sally, Laurel, John, Jim, and Barry.

Martin Donald for contributing his talents and passion for learning.

Joanne Coleman and Nick Nicholas for editing and encouragement.

Susan Smith for using her talents to teach us all.

Lucinda Wolinski, Cheri Smith, Colleen Jones and Mark Wolinski for continuing the belief.

Cynthia Franklin for welcoming me to this world and being the best "sister" ever.

And Terry McHenry for making every dream a reality.

LEARNING VICTORIES

This book is about you.
This book is about me.
It is about all learners.
We are all experiencing effort in
        acquiring,
        integrating
        and sharing information.
It is only a few rare learners
among us,
who master the confusion,
and experience learning as effortless.
I do not meet many of those persons
but I hear rumor
that they do exist.

Most learners experience stress in learning.
Some children experience considerable stress.
As children they are ravaged
by our educational systems.
Although some escape
with their self esteem intact,
most do not.
Some discover ways to alter their learning
to meet the demands of our educational
and work systems.
Others do not.
Some receive help
and understand their learning skills
and use them effectively.
They are the ones who have experienced -
Learning Victories.

FOREWORD

It was a shock to me when Dr. Joan Smith asked me to write the foreword to this book. I was shocked that she would perceive me as being capable of writing such a thing, especially for such an important book as this. In my heart, I was saying "Yes, yes, I want to do it. After all, I have benefitted from the teaching methods I've been exposed to thus far. I love the material in the manuscript I've read and can see how it could be beneficial to other people in many ways. The material is liberating. I do want to do this." I also had a lot of fear about it, and that's also, for me, a good indicator that it is a "must do" opportunity. So this is the way I write a foreword. I write it gratefully and admiringly for Dr. Joan Smith, whose work is brilliant, for a book that is invaluable, and with hope for many, many dear people, that they too will have the opportunity to experience their learning victories.

I have always avoided writing whenever possible not only because of the extreme difficulty felt in composing my thoughts but also because of the confusion as my thoughts would shoot off in every direction imaginable. And even if I could manage to pull this request together, get it down on paper in a fairly comprehensible form, it would never measure up to even *some* of the *real writers* of the world. An intelligent person, a real writer, can let thoughts gracefully flow from his/her uncluttered mind through open, creative channels to the fingers, while mentally plucking the perfect, tastiest words along the way to perfectly express a brilliant thought. And they can do it with the speed of light. I, on the other hand, would once again be chiseling a stone wheel for the journey.

I have revealed a few critical facts about my process. For one, I have been very critical...with myself. What I learned through Edu-Therapeutics is... don't be. I'm not perfect and neither is anyone else. Another fact is that writing this foreword is not a test; it is an exercise and an opportunity to challenge some fears I have. Edu-Therapeutics helped me with that. Another fact is that I had a misconception about my intelligence based on my poor academic performance due to my specific learning style. What I have learned is, and I loved these words, I have a specific dyslexic learning style. Now isn't that informative and hopeful at the same time? I think that just hearing that statement was my first victory. I don't have a handicap; my educators and the system in which I tried to learn had the handicap. Now there is a solution to that problem. In addition, because of the shame I felt due to misconceptions I had about my intelligence, and the secrecy I maintained because of my fear of being found out about my "handicap", I altered my life. My self expression was limited. Many of my questions were never constructed and asked, and I have had a lot of questions, ironically, because I have always loved learning. Edu-Therapeutics honors uniqueness and reveres the gifts and potential that uniqueness and diversity offer. I have learned that and at this very moment I am experiencing my uniqueness because of that kind of validation.

From the moment of accepting this request, my goal has been to let you know there is hope. I want you to know that more than anything I can think of. I don't care that you know me but that you know something of my experiences. It is not important to me that you think well of me as a writer but that you recognize, through my writing, the victory over some of my fear and shame. I think it is very important that you are aware of the tools, through Edu-Therapeutics, so that you too may create more victories in your life. I leave you with my deepest regrets for the pain you may have encountered and endured because of dyslexia. I also leave you with hope placed in your hands. Be inspired. Be you.

Martin Donald

TABLE OF CONTENTS

INTRODUCTION

This book introduces you to seven Victors! Each has experienced learning in a different manner and each has realized victories in minor and major ways.

Melody - Is a professional educator who realized that she shared the difficulty that many of her students experienced. She found it difficult to listen. She found that she labored over formulating her own thoughts and responses. She found that she was depressed much of the time and unsure about her intellectual skills.

Ron - A bartender and aspiring writer who started and stopped one career after another. He believed that he was inadequate in gaining information and that others easily learned what was so difficult for him. He wanted to learn quickly and easily but rarely experienced that he had achieved his goals.

Mark - A creative, artistic gentleman with major responsibility for a creative program who felt that he could not read to make sense of information. He knew that he would be experiencing a career change with an impending move and was fearful that his inefficiency in acquiring new information through reading would hamper his success.

Liz - A competent office administrator who found

herself falling apart when she attempted to extend her work horizons. The demands of a new position and learning new content areas brought back those fears and horrors that had followed her throughout her schooling.

Tim - a bank executive who found that his position of responsibility required more of his time management and organizational skills than he could assemble. He recognized that he could not share his knowledge in public forums and felt stymied to continue to advance in his chosen career. He wanted to develop his own business plan and had many talents in entrepreneurship.

Nancy - A nationally ranked athlete and personal trainer who found school a continually frustrating experience. She decided to confront her learning issues with personal effort and sheer fortitude. She used her knowledge of her unique dietary requirements and learning interventions to address the difficulty in learning that dyslexia visits upon the learner.

Lucy - A creative, bright youngster who has not learned to read or write despite years of special education assistance through her school. She is frustrated with learning. She specializes in avoiding school demands whenever possible. Her skills in avoiding educational experiences and her unique nutritional responses caused this gifted child to be labeled with *low-average* intelligence. She is to become the

Nancy, Liz, Melody, Ron, Tim or Mark of our next generation unless we can teach her to become a victor in learning.

In our adventure in learning we have found six areas which, in combination, will make a difference in the learning skills of our learners. We will understand the misbelief of our learners, that everyone else is **perfect** and only they are flawed. The misconception of perfection runs rampant through each of our learner's lives.

We found that all of our learners experienced difficulty in their attention processing and that their success in controlling their diets often paralleled their learning success. We learned that using imagery was a critical element in gaining control of their learning. We discovered that the issue of listening and comprehending what is being heard created havoc in their understanding. Each of these understandings and steps for resolution provided the movement along the way toward *learning victories.*

We were grateful that each of these learners was willing to share their experiences, frustrations and victories with us for this book. It is always much easier to recognize the commonalities in learning when we can listen to someone else's experiences. Learning is a genuine adventure with all of the incumbent disasters, frustrations, joys and hoped-for successes to be discovered in our journeys.

Chapter One

LEARNING AT ITS BEST

The most exciting element in working with our learners is that they are all highly intelligent. Several were fearful and guarded in expressing their frailties. The rest were curious and vulnerable. Yet each of them was open and willing to share the journey of learning that brought them to be seeking a *difference* in their learning.

There were several characteristics which each of the learners had in common. The first is **intellectual level**. These are all very bright people! Several have superior vocabularies with which they create an impression of confidence and competence. Several are bold and assertive in the way that they communicate. They are often amusing and display an apparent comfort in controlling conversations.

No one would ever suspect that, in fact, this was their way of avoiding listening and risking confusion in following what they were hearing.

Some of our learners were quiet and appeared to be reflective as they considered each situation or comment carefully before responding. They are gentle individuals who appear to have a quiet confidence. Yet they will describe this confidence as "pre-panic"! They are terrified that they will be asked to respond or perform in a manner in which they will make a mistake. Their fear has cost them greatly in emotional energy and has limited many of their choices. They are often depressed and fearful of being worthless.

The second characteristic they shared was a **drive for perfection**. In a perfect educational environment, these learners would have been directed to their strengths. They would have been celebrated for their abilities and guided in developing those areas which were not natural gifts in learning. We have yet to find this perfect world. So, each of our learners found that their parents, siblings and teachers combined to make their inefficiencies, errors and imperfections apparent. The emphasis in learning was, in fact, on identifying errors in thinking, in responding and in producing. The emphasis was on the need for the totally acceptable performance only - the perfect performance. Their identity as unique learners was undervalued and overlooked.

The result of these learning experiences was to de-emphasize the gifts and talents of each learner and to emphasize the vulnerabilities, inefficiencies and errors. The emphasis was on creating perfection. Ironically, the brighter the learners the more sensitive they were to having their suspected imperfections revealed. Each of the learners feared that someone would discover that they were imperfect. Many of them shared that this was what kept them from seeking help for their perceived problems. They were afraid that if they admitted their errors or vulnerability that they would be unworthy of what they had achieved. They were afraid of losing family, friends or jobs. They spent considerable energy daily in covering for their perceived differences.

The third characteristic each possessed was **confusion in listening.** They explained that they were constantly unsure if what they heard was really what was being said.

This confusion extended to listening to their own voices when they read. They were consistently confused with comprehension in reading and felt that they were not remembering what they were reading. The combination of difficulty in listening and reading comprehension created fear and doubt about their adequacy in understanding.

The reading comprehension confusion did not display itself in lowered reading test scores. Several of the learners could score above a high school level on comprehension tests. When they read a page of technical information, they found that they were unable to take in the details. Since they were filled with self-doubt, the problems were compounded as soon as they began to experience a loss of information.

Speeded-up processing [hyper-processing] was the fourth characteristic that each of our learners displayed. When they attempted to read information or respond they tended to do so very rapidly. They appeared to equate speed with success. Of course, the result of performance in "hyper-speed" was that they missed information. This compounded their confusion both for listening and reading comprehension.

It appeared that the fast attempts at working were part of the perception that speed equaled success. When someone responded rapidly to a comment, others would assume that they were intelligent. There also appeared to be a confusion about the processing of time. Therefore, there was little knowledge about acceptable amounts of time in waiting for a response. Everything had to be immediate.

The speeded-up processing was closely related to the fifth characteristic of most of the learners, **delayed response time**. Initially it appeared to be a contradiction of the fourth characteristic. But actually, it was very much connected, if not actually causative. Most of our learners tested as having a delay in their response time for processing stimuli. This specific type of attention disorder was very confusing for them. It created a lag between the time that a stimulus was received and an accurate and adequate response could be formulated.

The delay appeared to incite within the learner a need to increase the speed in responses. The learners experienced a feeling that they needed to *hurry-up* to perform acceptably. They frequently seized the opportunity to respond rapidly by inserting irrelevant or inappropriate comments.

They were often aware of *blurting-out* a comment and wishing that they had not done so. They found themselves interrupting the normal flow of conversation by inserting unrelated comments. Since they were unable to process the incoming information appropriately they usually had little idea of the responses that they should be providing. As we shall observe, this response time issue was most likely the major component in their frustration in learning.

Finally, each of our learners shared a challenge in using their **visual imagery**. Two of the learners actually recalled having made a conscious decision to shut it off. It appeared that they were very visual and it distracted them from listening. They believed as children that they would do better if they ignored it and so they did. For each of our learners, this was a major issue. They did not easily image information nor did they

8

believe that they could.

A lack of imagery seriously complicates one's ability to experience comprehension. It is especially important in reading descriptive information such as history, novels or classical literature. To miss the joy of having a story or a scene come-alive in one's mind is a great loss. It also impacts on listening to descriptive information and can create considerable confusion, as we will hear from our learners. Fortunately, the skill can be developed and, with the efforts each learner exerted, imagery again became a reality for them.

These six characteristics are important elements in the learning style for dyslexic and/or attention-stressed individuals. The identification, isolation and intervention for each of these characteristics was key in the success of each of our learners. As we journey with them in their search for a solution for the stresses they experience in learning, we will find that we all experience some of these issues every day.

Chapter Two

ATTRIBUTES OF LEARNING

All learners share the same attributes of learning. It is the combination of *strengths* and *inefficiencies* within each attribute which makes each of us different in our learning abilities. It is the balance between our attributes which enables us to be skilled or challenged in a particular area.

The attributes which are used in our system of Edu-Therapeutics have been simplified to include nine areas:

INTELLIGENCE

Intelligence may be the collective label that includes all of our attributes. It relies on memory, creativity, attention, concept formation and skills in executive function and, undoubtedly, many more. It is often observable, even when it is not measurable. Our skills in measuring intelligence are still very primitive. The appearance of intelligence as an attribute is dependent upon many factors including, as we see with Lucy, nutrition.

CREATIVITY

Creativity is the ability to say, see or do something in a unique

10

way. It is the skill of putting together uncommon elements in a way that is successful or pleasing to the creator. It is a totally subjective attribute and one of the most fragile and vulnerable of our attributes. It is truly sensitive to external and internal feedback and easily nurtured or destroyed during our early learning years.

ATTENTION

There are two variables that are important in attention: time and screening. Time is related to how long [*duration*] we can attend to something. Time often varies depending upon the stimulus which is being received. Individuals with time confusion often have difficulty in monitoring the passing of time, and have minimal conceptualization about how long it takes to do something.

Screening refers to the ability we have to direct our attention toward, or ignore, the stimuli around us. It refers to the ability to control our attention related to our internal stimuli [*inner voice* or *visualizations*] and the external stimuli from our environment.

VISUAL MEMORY

Most of us experience skill in our visual imagery for concrete or *experienced* images. We can recognize the house we live

11

in or family members at the most basic level.

Recalling a sequence of unrelated symbols is more difficult for many of us. This skill is required for reading and spelling. The subtle variation in the symbols which create changes in the appearance between a cursive "a ", printed "A" or typed "a" are often confusing.

Visual memory provides us with the foundation for our visualizations. It enables us to recognize familiar elements or to recreate images with our *seen* inner language.

AUDITORY MEMORY

Listening skills are often difficult for individuals with dyslexic or attention-related learning styles. When this attribute is inefficient it creates considerable difficulty in learning. Listening to information which provides related content is often easier than retaining unrelated or sequential information. It is easier to recall hearing that Joe's house is green with purple shutters than that his house number is located at 24983 Sheridan Way.

When language relates information together it is far easier to recall. Unrelated information such as phone numbers or formulas are more difficult. It is our auditory memory which is essential for registering the sequence of phonemes (sound units) in language and for comprehension.

Auditory memory is important in receiving both what others tell us and what we are thinking ourselves. We have all experienced wanting to tell someone something we were just thinking about, but forgetting it once we opened our mouths. Our working auditory memory is stressed by emotional issues, nutrition, health (fatigue or stress) and lack of experience or use. It can be developed effectively with intervention and conscious intent to expand it.

TIME ORIENTATION
AND CONCEPTUALIZATION

Understanding where we are in time is an essential attribute for planning, organizing and implementing our executive function [*strategy*] skills. It is crucial to understand the time-organization of a week, a month, a year, a course of study, a vacation, etc.

It is equally important to have a concept about how long it takes to do something. If we do not understand that it takes only minutes to brush our teeth, we may continually put it off because we do not have time. If we think it will take hours and hours to do a homework assignment of writing ten spelling words three times each, we may avoid it as long as possible.

13

Appropriate conceptualization of time issues are critical for learning. It often requires specific intervention and effort to develop this concept, but because of its importance, the impact on a learner's productivity is very positive.

AUDITORY CONCEPTUALIZATION

When we hear or read a description of a scene, we can enjoy it if we are able to visualize it. This attribute enables us to take what we hear and register it as both a verbal and visual image. It relies primarily on effective reception of the auditory input. The visual image is then matched or constructed based on the detail of auditory information received.

Auditory conceptualization is reading comprehension. It is the ability to listen to our inner language, read a story and to match visual images, to create a scene, character or event.

VISUAL CONCEPTUALIZATION

Visual conceptualization is the *flip side* of auditory conceptualization. It is the ability to see something and to register or record it with words.

It is important in communication. It is the ability to describe what happened, what one saw, or to communicate to another person, what our brain has registered as information.

MOTORIC SKILLS

A motor skill is the ability to coordinate movements to accomplish a specific goal. It may be the ability to move our fingers with a pencil and write legibly, to kick a football, or to type a letter. It is any motor skill which requires a complex sequence of movements.

When we think of learning as requiring specific attributes, we look at each learner as being unique. This is the basis for therapy with Edu-Therapeutics. Therapists and teachers trained in Edu-Therapeutics are able to identify the attributes the learner possesses. When we use this learning system, we can recognize the efficiency level in using an attribute. From this understanding we can choose the solutions for developing efficiency in learning.

Our first focus will be on intelligence. It is important for us to recognize that it is, in fact, an attribute which impacted our learners. Obviously it is an attribute to celebrate. Few of them had experienced that option before, and they came to enjoy the comfort of knowing that they had the **power to learn**.

Chapter Three

THE BURDEN OF INTELLECT

"You are bright, you can do it." This seemed to be the theme song most of our learners shared. Beginning in their early school years, parents and teachers frequently told them, "You can do it, just TRY." In fact, they heard it so frequently, they believed that they were guilty of "not trying."

They each experienced the frustration of an inability to accomplish at the level everyone expected. Very rapidly the frustration was replaced with a *fear*. They were afraid that their teachers and parents would discover that they really were not *intelligent* after all. They were fearful of losing the status and assurance of being *bright!*

The longer each learner experienced inabilities to understand information or perform to a standard, the more the fear grew. The fear became a suspicion that if they were not bright they were *stupid* ! The fear became *shame* and *terror* in learning.

Only very intelligent minds have the capacity for analysis

which these learners possess. At very early ages they identified the discrepancy between what they were supposed to learn and what they learned. They registered the subtle differences between what others in the class were doing, and what they were doing. They recorded what their teachers said to them and analyzed it for every possible clue as to their worth. They internalized comments, criticisms and statements which reflected on their value or worth from every significant person in their youth.

> *Beginning in kindergarten, the teacher told my parents that I was different. They were very concerned about me. I could tell by their whispered confidences after every talk with the teacher.*

> *I have gone back and read my report cards from those grades. The teachers in the first three grades told my parents I was "slow". Even though they were both teachers themselves, they believed my teachers. They treated me kindly and constantly helped me with my work. Mother was always there to give me assistance. I knew something must be very wrong.*

> *I did not seem to have many friends by third grade. I liked to read. I read the newspaper every day after school. I listened to my parents discuss issues but I knew I should not be in the conversation.*

17

This incredibly-bright individual was brought to us when he was twenty-two and living at home. His parents were frightened that he was slow and would never be able to hold a job. He had accepted this image of himself. I started by asking him for evidence that he was *slow*. He referred to the report cards (which he kept in his top drawer and read frequently!).

I told him that we were going to establish evidence that the report cards were *lies* and then he was going to put them away forever. We looked at his academic scores on his current testing. We looked at his early ability to read and retain and analyze information. We discussed the attributes he had, that enabled him to do those tasks.

We talked about his parent's *confusion* and the *error* they made in believing one teacher instead of trusting their own observations. We discussed that our parents are not perfect and they can only do what they think is best at the time. His mother verbalized to him [with considerable coaching] that she believed now that the teacher had made an error. With this admission, his mother gave him back his intellectual power and let go of her need to protect him. Now, at the age of twenty-four, he runs his own landscape business and is married.

If he had not been bright, he would not have realized what was happening to him. He would not have been sensitive to how he was being treated differently. He might not have responded in the way that was being prescribed for him....*act slow, be dependent, need help!*

Ron, a bartender and writer, is a brilliant individual with an incredible vocabulary. He provided a marvelous description of what it is like to be incredibly bright and *fragmented!*

> *My ideas are like wild horses in my mind. I have to lasso them to get them, to be able to think. I work to slow my mind down and gain control.*

His verbal skills are astounding. He can speak on many subjects with great ease and strong content. He loves being creative and developing stories with ironic or amusing twists in them. In one of his plays he wrote...

> *There is this man and he is walking around in the library and he comes to the mystery section. He pulls out a book, it looks like a rather new book, and he turns toward the last few pages and he rips them out. He stuffs them in his pocket and puts the book back on the shelf.*
>
> *The next scene takes place in the lobby of the library. An old man is walking, practically running, to the person at the information desk, saying "I checked this mystery book*

19

out, a week ago, and the last few pages are torn out. I don't know who did it but I am very angry." The clerk is kind of flustered, and he says, "Well, I'm very sorry. Let me get you the librarian, Mr. Bender. There he is, Mr. Bender..."

The camera pans to the same man who was walking around in the mystery section in the beginning. The old man is quite irate and yelling at Mr. Bender. Mr. Bender says to the man, "Well, I'm really sorry about this. We will order a new copy. In the meantime we just got this new book in, you might want to read it." And he hands the man the book he had just ripped the pages out of....

Ron was in his teens when he realized that he experienced a different way of learning from his peers.

JS -When did you decide that you had some differences in your learning, that you were unique in your learning?

R - You are so non-judgmental in all of your words, it's incredible.

JS -They are differences really... did you register them emotionally or intellectually?

R - Well, emotionally, that happened a long time ago. Probably when I was still in my teens, maybe or before that. I think my personality changed because of that or developed because of it. Anyway that is something I can just guess at. But intellectually it was in the 80's, probably about a decade ago, when that happened.

JS - Where were you in your life at that time? Were you in school?

R - I am sure I was. I was in and out of school my entire life but whether or not I was in, really, I don't know. I had already graduated from college with my BS and that was in the 70's. So it had to be later. I came across a couple of words, dyslexia was one. It's going to seem absurd to you, its absurd to me now. Now I realize , I don't have these things, but you have to understand I was grasping for something, for some understanding. I heard words like aphasia. I said, "Hey, that's me, I don't understand what I read." That was when it first started happening. I had this analogy about something that was wrong.

JS - Can you share it?

R - It was like a hose, a garden hose with a kink in it and water. If there is no kink in the hose the water flows out smoothly, but if you put a kink in it, it starts coming out all over the place. I began to think that maybe that was the problem. I was doing all of these things to try and figure out what the problem was. I never did, but I felt I ought to.

21

JS - So in college you were really on track and did not have any difficulties that caused you to work harder.

R - Well, I developed a way, unconsciously, at an early age, of handling school. I've always put off studying to the last minute. It reminds me of the quotes from one of the poets from the book on attention disorders. It's something about a man who says, the night before he is going to be hanged..."It clears the mind." For years now I have had the feeling that my mind has been sluggish and it takes a feeling of real anxiety..gee, I've got to get this done... or I won't even start it. I won't even think about it until then.

The way I have studied is to goof off in class. Taking notes in class is just like the list you asked me to write, which I did not do, because I do not know how to write it. I don't know what is important or isn't important. When I start thinking about that list, I started to think...I've got to write this down...there were six or seven subsets of that. The list would have been so long I would have missed work while I was working on the list!

That's the way notes have always been for me. I never knew what was important to take down. So, I think at an early age, long before I realized I was doing it, I would goof off in class because I was good verbally. I was good at getting laughs. Then I would study at the last minute. I would get somebody else's notes and study off them.

JS - Did you make sense of them?

R - Of the notes? That's a very good question, I made sense of them enough to pass the test, but I never ever thought about if I could remember, or make sense to the point that I would internalize, it so that it would stay there. You know what I mean?

JS - I am intrigued that you could pick up someone else's notes and pass a test with them?

R - Geez, I could do it far better than I could with my notes! I was in a journalism class and we had to take information from a worksheet with several paragraphs and organize it into a lead paragraph. I couldn't organize the information. So I asked the other old gentleman in the class to work together. We worked together, but we didn't actually work together. He organized the information. I wrote my own paragraph and he wrote his own paragraph. I got the highest grade in the class. It was a very difficult class, but that is only in part because I knew how to use notes.

The other gentleman got mad at me. He couldn't write the leads as effectively as I could. But he could organize the information. I remember thinking, I was kind of arrogantly thinking,...Gee, Look at this, I wrote these leads and got an excellent grade... But yet, how can I be a writer or a journalist when I couldn't organize the

23

information. I could go out and get it, but I couldn't organize it. So I knew then that something was lacking as well...and it sort of hit home.

It was one of the little epiphanies that I remember throughout my life. It was one of those things that I couldn't organize this information, no matter how important it was to me and I realized I didn't realize it. Actually, I am just realizing it now. I am unable to take the information I get in a classroom and sift through it and put it in a place or position where I can use it later on.

*For a long time I have called myself spontaneous and I told you one time I am a **prisoner of spontaneity**. Ideas just fly about and I say them. I can't stop thinking of new ideas to do the boring stuff.*

The attributes of intelligence are certainly complemented by an ability to be spontaneous, and creative. Ron shares quite vividly the feeling of being trapped with his intelligent mind. Coupled with his inefficiencies in several attributes of processing, including time management, auditory conceptualization and visual conceptualization, his intellect has created doubt and pain.

A different type of intelligence is apparent with Tim. He is an entrepreneur. He is constantly developing new projects which will make money. His mind races in a different direction than Ron's but is obviously performing *with uncontrolled speed*! He can easily relate to the "wild horses" description. He is also very

24

verbal. His expertise is in salesmanship. He is in the banking business and consistently develops successful new programs and marketing plans for his branch. He wants to leave his job and have his own business but is unable to organize himself to accomplish this goal.

> *I am afraid to tell anyone about my latest business plan. I know that it is sound but it seems that every time I tell someone they poke holes in it and I give it up. I don't think I will talk about it anymore. It is too frustrating to keep starting over.*

When Tim works within the structure of his position in the bank, his ideas can be effectively implemented. He wants to be independent of this structure and use his own resources, his intellect, for his own goals. His intelligence allows him to see the opportunities for success but his challenge in processing and time management continually foil his efforts and leave him vulnerable.

Lucy is a very bright fifth grader. She has been in resource classes at school since second grade. When she first came to us, she was unable to read. We are using Edu-Therapeutics with her and increasing her skills in her learning attributes.

The key factor related to Lucy's learning is that she experiences a slow response time. Her response time appears to be related to what she eats. When she has a restricted diet her skills change dramatically.

During her fifth grade year, Lucy was re-evaluated by the school psychologist. He identified that she had "lower end of the average" intelligence. In the report he noted that her full scale dropped markedly from the 105 recorded three years ago but that her performance scores remained fairly consistent.

The assessment that was administered was the Wechsler Intelligence Scale for Children - III. The scores which are reported with each subtest are on a scale of 1-20 with an average score of 10. Intelligence is reported on a scale with an average of 100 with scores in the 130's indicating gifted skills. These are the scores from her assessment:

Wechsler Intelligence Scale for Children			
Verbal Subtests		Performance Subtests	
Information	9	Picture Completion	6
Similarities	8	Coding	13
Arithmetic	7	Picture Arrangement	11
Vocabulary	8	Block Design	10
Comprehension	9	Object Assembly	8
Verbal IQ	90	Performance IQ	98
	Full Scale I.Q. 93		

We were aware that Lucy was very bright. It is obvious that her response time has confounded her ability to respond on her testing.

During one session, Lucy wanted to work with the Tower of Hanoi (a manipulation exercise using rings which increase in size and are placed on a post on a platform with three posts. The task is to move the rings from one post to another post without placing a larger ring on a smaller ring.) She was very unfocused and could not do the task. She started hiding the pieces under her chair and generally distracting herself from the task.

The next day, Lucy returned for her lesson and asked to again work with the Tower. I was not very excited about repeating this experience again and stipulated that she must first complete all her other work. To my surprise she did her work quickly and had plenty of time for her choice activity.

I sat in total amazement as Lucy manipulated the rings on the posts in the minimum amount of moves and concluded the task with confidence. When I asked her how she had accomplished this, she reported, "I thought about it in the middle of the night and it came to me!"

Adults have difficulty doing this task. Lucy, an eleven year old with a slightly below average IQ, did it by thinking about it during the night. I shared these observations

> *with her mother and we agreed that we would repeat her*
> *intelligence test after an appropriate amount of time had*
> *lapsed. We also agreed that we would monitor her diet for*
> *two weeks prior to the testing.*

Lucy's second assessment, after an appropriate delay to avoid issues of familiarity with the test items, was administered with startling results. The most amazing aspect of the assessment was her concentration and focus.

Wechsler Intelligence Scale for Children III			
Verbal Subtests		Performance Subtests	
Information	9	Picture Completion	10
Similarities	15	Coding	11
Arithmetic	8	Picture Arrangement	19
Vocabulary	9	Block Design	18
Comprehension	14	Object Assembly	15
Verbal I.Q.	106	Performance I.Q.	131
	Full Scale I.Q.	120	

Not only was Lucy's overall score considerably different [over one standard deviation above the previous score] but her performance was equally astounding. She performed far beyond her scores in either test during the prior six years. She was fast and on-target on each task.

It is important to understand that Lucy did not change in some of the areas. The areas which were not improved by her dietary adjustment were those which required listening skills to gain information. During these years of school Lucy has not been *clear and present* in her attention and reception. This is a phenomena which occurs in learning. Even though we have a very intelligent brain, if we are not inputting information efficiently, our I.Q. scores will drop. We have not lost intelligence. We have missed out on content [information] which is measured during the assessment.

Any of the areas in which Lucy could use her own skills to adjust to the task were successful for her. Tasks in which she had to have specific content information, such as knowledge of arithmetic facts or vocabulary, did not change because the information simply was missing. For instance, one question asks "What is a fable?". Lucy had no idea what a fable was and could not recall ever hearing about it.

Many of Lucy's learning challenges are associated with her slow response time. We will look at her attention skills and this important attribute in a subsequent chapter.

Attribute training can alter our ability to perform effectively on intelligence tests. Change will be observed over a period of time. It does not occur in a few months time but it can occur in a year. When children or adults appear to be intelligent but are having difficulty in performing effectively, we must look at their attributes and identify where the

29

inefficiencies are located. By developing the attribute skills in the areas of inefficiency, we provide the learner with extended resources to use in learning.

Each of the individuals featured in this collection has unique attribute profiles which reflect their intellectual powers. They were not selected because they were unusual but because they are *representative* of learners who experience attention and/or dyslexic learning styles. During the past thirty years we have evaluated over ten thousand individuals at the *Melvin-Smith Learning Centers* and this is the consistent profile that we see.

They frequently share with us that everyone says they are "bright" and they quietly share their fear that they are really "dumb"! Who would expect that being *bright* could be such a *burden.*

Chapter Four

PERFECTIONISM
A SERIOUS CHALLENGE

Webster's New World Dictionary tells us that *perfect* means "complete in all respects, flawless,...excellent as in skills or quality... completely accurate." Being perfect is an apparent goal in much of our culture. Unfortunately it undermines the confidence of, otherwise, effective and successful individuals. Being perfect assumes that there is a single, specific way of performing and responding that is acceptable to everyone, everywhere, at all times. When we perform in that manner we are perfect.

There are two types of perfectionism that we encounter frequently:

1. Perfection as defined by a significant adult (teacher or parent) in our early years and built-in as an expectation.
2. Perfection as defined by our own observations of difference from others, creating an assumption that we are flawed because of the difference.

This definition of *perfection* is especially significant for our intelligent students and adults who have experienced a learning inefficiency or unique learning style. Instead of being able to focus on their effective skills and talents, they seem to magnify their differences as imperfections. Unfortunately, this choice seems to occur at a very early age. Usually it occurs about the time the individual enters school and meets the initial frustration in conforming to what he or she observes others doing. Since this belief is established so early, it becomes an integral part of our belief system about ourselves.

The impact of perfectionism on learning is significant. It is especially an issue for bright, creative learners. Whenever they encounter frustration, they assume that it is their fault because they are basically flawed in some way. This was well illustrated with Melody's reaction to difficulty in learning a new skill in her work.

> *Melody - I feel like I should be staying at lower levels so that I can get all the information.*

> *JS - Lower means what to you?*

> *M - I am having trouble remembering the words and the content. I can repeat what they say but when I start to understand it, I forget what they are saying.*

> *JS - An awful lot of that is normal response to stress.*

> *M - I just wanted to check on it.*

JS - There are very few people who automatically retain every detail. It is not part of the normal human condition. We are very imperfect and our brains are asked to not just be listening but processing... What is going on here? What am I really getting? Is it really true? In addition, our brain is helping us maintain an upright position, not falling over, and so many things at once. It is trying to screen out who is walking by and who is answering the phone. If we could totally isolate ourselves and not have to do anything except listen and image with our eyes shut with no stimuli around us, we would be likely to be more perfect in doing only one thing at a time. That is not what we have to do. What standards do you think you will be held to?

M - I don't know.

JS - Why don't you inquire, because the standard you are assuming appears to be perfection.

M - That could be mine, my interpretation of it because I ask, require, that of myself. I am working on it. I am getting a lot better about not being perfect but I still think that maybe I need to be doing better and I am failing.

JS - Remember yesterday in our discussion, I shared with you that perfectionism tends to go with brightness. The more intelligent the person the more they think they should-a, ought-a get every detail...because they have very bright, alert minds and they processes a lot and they want it all.

M - I see other people processing differently than I do, so I take it...

JS - They are better than you?

M - Well, no (guilty laugh), no, I don't think so.

JS - This is an interesting phenomenon. Everyone with whom I have worked on this particular series tells me that everyone else does better than they do. They see it and, therefore, they know.

M - Well, I see them doing it.

JS - Doing what?

M - Well, there is this woman at work who thinks really well about things. She evaluates things very well. And I don't do that well. I don't know, but I make assumptions, usually wrong assumptions based upon what it is or what I thought it is.

JS - And what is the image that these thoughts create for you about yourself?

M - It's rotten.

At this point Melody made the shift and began to work with the impact of her perfectionism. It was essential to reach this point in her exploration because we could put it up for discussion.

> *JS - What is the image you create for yourself when you are focusing on what you do right ?*
>
> *M - That I am capable and doing well.*
>
> *JS - What is the image you project to others?*
>
> *M - That I am very capable.*
>
> *JS - You brought an interesting person to me this week. I have seen a person who is bright and capable. This person asks good questions and is inquisitive beyond the normal person. Why do you suppose this person is constantly punishing herself because she is not perfect? You have very high standards and the ability to measure your performance in detail. As a matter of fact, you measure everything and compare it to your standard. Unfortunately, when you get eighty percent of the information, you are moaning because you got twenty percent wrong! Instead, you could choose to be saying, "I got eighty percent right, I did a good job."*
>
> *M - But...*
>
> *JS - Oops, here comes the Perfection-Standards Cop!*

> *A lot of this comes from our childhood. I am a lot older than you, but in my era, there was a strong belief in parenting that you had to point out to the child the errors that they were making so that they could correct them. And the good parents were the ones who made the differentiation and pointed it out....a lot!*

> *M - That's what I grew up with.*

Melody experienced the standards that were defined by her teachers and her parents. The expectation was for her to be successful in the attributes which were valued at that time. Since she was very bright, she internalized those standards and adopted them for herself. Whenever she saw that she was not measuring up to the high standards, she felt that she was *flawed.* She assumed responsibility for those standards and they governed all of her expectations.

We are all a product of the messages we receive in our early years. The balance point between acceptance and encouragement to achieve to greater standards is impossibly sensitive. It is one that is extremely difficult to establish for students with consistent learning skills. Students with inefficiencies in learning, are even greater challenges with this balance point to their parents and teachers. This is because observations which are available regarding their learning skills create confusion. In some tasks they are superior and at

36

ease. On other tasks they experience great confusion and frustration.

Initially parents and teachers assume that the student is lazy or not trying. This is because they are obviously intelligent and *obviously not succeeding.* Pressure in many forms is used to attempt to *motivate* the student to be effective. In fact, most of us internalize the messages of the *Critic Voice.* The messages we have heard about what we *should or ought to* be doing are recorded in our critic voice and embedded in our long-term memory.

If our learners *could* they *would.* It is very uncomfortable for them to experience the irritation and disappointment of parents and teachers. The more pressure they register, the more panicked they become, and the less effective they are in resolving their confusion.

> *M - I am trying to get to change myself but it is so hard.*

> *JS - It makes no sense but it is the way we are. We need to move on. Whenever we have the feeling that we are not going to be successful, in other words perfect, it tightens us up. We immediately bring out our Critic and replay the old-lecture about being perfect. Then we are certain to make the errors we*

are afraid of because we are focusing on them and giving ourselves negative messages.

M - I do that.

JS - Everyone does that.   When we are focusing on the error or the difficulty, instead of the image of completing it correctly, we have only one choice, and that is to make the error. We need to allow our brain to relax, to focus on the process of completing the task and allow ourselves to use our energy to achieve the goal.   I shared with you our experience in working with people with head injuries.   They often start to have their memories return while they are sleeping, in their dreams, when they are totally relaxed.   We should take a cue from this knowledge. We need to release ourselves from the pressure, relax and enjoy the process of finding a solution or completing a task.

Not everyone has to get all of their information from visualizing it.   Sometimes it is just as good to remember what we are hearing. Sometimes we have snatches of both! We are not imperfect if we choose to use one learning skill or attribute or another. Certain tasks call for specific attributes or can be done with many different attributes. We want to be flexible in how we use our attributes and enjoy using

38

them. We won't be perfect and we don't have to be!

M - So its okay if I don't do it the same as others do?

JS - You got the message. Viva la difference! Wouldn't it be boring if we were all the same and there was only one way to do everything?

M - So I don't have to image everything perfectly?

JS - Good grief, what a cluttered mind we would have if we tried to image everything. Let's relax, take a breath, let all of our senses enjoy the experience. And we won't be perfect and we don't have to be!

Over the years it has become apparent to me that there is no *perfect person*. I have met many individuals who have amazing talents in specific (and a few in many) areas. Although they were very accomplished, none of them was perfect in every way. In fact, most of them would elucidate their shortcomings with great frequency. It has always astounded me how ready we are to point out our inefficiencies and be critical about ourselves.

The result of feeling that we need to be perfect or *right* is to experience *panic*. Whenever we perceive that we are not being totally successful, such as when we experience stress in receiving or processing, we feel panicky. Throughout the sessions with each of our learners the discussion of panic or fear has been an important theme. This was a common characteristic of both male and female learners. When they experienced a challenge with a task, they panicked. It is essential to contradict this reaction pattern and replace it with one of comfort.

Since the process of therapy involves stretching the individuals to the edge of their skill, we consistently evoked the panic response. This was done purposefully. If everything that the learner was asked to do was comfortable and easy then they would quickly assume that we did not understand their needs and issues. It is important, as we say during the sessions, " *to dangle you on the edge of confusion.*" We always tell the learners that understanding their edge communicates that we know where their skills are functioning. During each session we teach new skills and *stretch the edge further.* Tasks which were impossible during an early session are simple later in the process.

Panic is actually a fear. It is the fear that there is a loss of control. By teaching our learners how to regain their learning control they can eliminate the panic response. There are times when panic is a health reaction. As we discussed during one of the sessions, panic usually stimulates an adrenalin response. This is akin to the *flight or fight* response. Neither of these is particularly useful in learning. It does, however, explain why learners often want to run away from a learning experience or become angry.

Mark - This Figural Mind Bender is difficult. I can't find the right position for the shape. See, my mind is already wandering. It can't be this because... Don't say anything. It won't go right there. Can I say something? I feel it for a moment and then I lose it. I want to run away and hide. I feel scared.

JS - That is a common reaction to confusion. You will feel like taking a deep breath and a drink of your water. You will want to start conditioning yourself that it is okay to have this feeling. You can acknowledge the feeling. Tell me more about it. Let's get to know the feeling.

M - It is inside me. I feel like I am all shaking inside.

JS - Let's tell ourselves that it is a message that we need to look at other choices and other solutions. It is a feeling we can let go of so that we can stay focused on the process of finding a solution. Would you like to say to yourself that you register the feeling? (Nod). Now say that you are in control and the feeling you experienced is only a message. You

41

are not controlled by the message. You get to choose.

M - I have been doing that more and more. When I start to panic, I say "Eh, its okay". Hey, I have it. I think I solved the problem. Lets check my answer. As soon as I let go, the answer came to me!

We need to change our internal language as we talk to ourselves. We can be our own guides in talking our way to a solution. One of the key words we use in helping learners enjoy the process of gaining new skills is to *experiment*. We ask them to *experiment* with this task. This word evokes an entirely different set of expectations during the learning process. We are no longer attempting to find *the answer* or be perfect. We are using a process to find an answer. We are experimenting with different ways of solving the problem.

Everyone knows that not all experiments are going to be successful. That is why it is an experiment. When we start to experiment with writing a paper, studying for a test, solving a mind-bender problem, we focus on the process, not the result. This is where we want our learners focused.

The second part of experimenting is that it is *fun*. We want to make learning fun, challenging and thought provoking. This is a pleasant experience. Learning needs to be a pleasant experience.

Melody - You want me to memorize all these pictures and then tell them to you? (Nod) How many are there? Twelve?

JS - What is that look you are giving me.

M - I doubt if I can do that. I might miss some.

JS - You might not be perfect?

M - No, well, I guess that is what I am saying.

JS - We are going to do this differently. We are going to experiment with ways to learn these. You know about an experiment. It is trying things out. [Nod] Will they all work?

M - No, not if I am doing them.

JS -You and everyone else. All learning is an experiment. It is trying different ways of gaining information and seeing if we retain and can apply it.

M - Are you serious? That sounds too easy. It sounds comfortable.

JS - It is comfortable and so is learning. We just have

> *to experiment with different strategies until we find the one we want to use in this situation. Then we use it!*

The concept of experimenting removes the expectation of knowing *the answer*. We all seem to assume that everyone else knows the answer and we are the only ones who have to work at it. Working at it is part of our brain process. Most of us have to work at learning, work at solving problems and work at gaining new skills. Our perfectionists assume that they are the only ones who have to suffer in learning. They believe that for everyone else it is easy and automatic. It is important for every learner to understand that, even if they do not talk about it in general conversation, everyone must work at certain types of learning.

Perfectionism is a serious issue. It creates failures. It stimulates panic and fear. It blocks learners from being successful. We can successfully control the Critic within by providing ourselves with new messages. We can focus on the process and experiment with finding the answer and the solution. We can remove the fear and regain the fun of learning.

Chapter Five

CONFUSION IN LISTENING

The major issue each of our learners experienced was a confusion in listening. This is the most difficult of the attributes to understand and to accommodate. It is usually misidentified as related to behavioral or emotional issues.

The listening confusion may have several possible sources. It may be related to inadequate auditory processing memory skill, difficulty with auditory discrimination or a delay in processing speed.

Auditory Memory: This skill enables us to recall what we hear and retain the order (sequence) of the information. By the time a child is eight years old, he or she can recall a sequence of six digits with reasonable consistency. An adult would find ease in memory with a recall of seven to eight digits.

Auditory Discrimination: An awareness of the subtle differences in sounds is important in understanding speech and aiding in spelling. It may be complicated by subtle or significant hearing issues.

Processing Delay: Current research is showing

that there may be an actual delay in milliseconds in a learner's ability to register the sounds he is hearing.

The difficulty in identifying auditory processing skills is imbedded in our educational system's awareness of this issue. Since students with this inefficiency tend to *appear* to be *not listening* or not trying to learn, it is this behavioral observation to which we respond. The student is usually admonished to "pay attention", or is punished for "not trying".

Many of the students who are identified as having an *attention disorder* actually have auditory processing inefficiencies. Some experience both. It is very important to differentiate between attention deficit disorder and auditory processing confusion before providing treatment or therapy.

The confusion which exists in auditory processing has a significant impact on the learner. Since it is so often misunderstood, learners receive confusing messages from parents and teachers. The emotional baggage associated with this particular learning inefficiency is often significant. The reason for the impact is that the learner does not receive verbal messages effectively. Therefore, learners attempt to *fill-in the message* with what they *think* is being said.

During my first year of teaching I had a specific demonstration of the impact and frustration of

46

auditory confusion. Frank, a nice young man in my learning handicapped class was playing on the school yard with a bat and ball. He was tossing the ball in the air and hitting it, and then chasing it himself.

A group of sixth graders decided to tease him and when he hit the ball, they ran after it and threw it away from him. He continued to pursue it and they played "keep-a-way." When the yard teacher saw the incident she called the students in to admonish them. The sixth graders claimed that he had been chasing them with the bat and they were running from him, because he was trying to hit them.

Of course, the entire group ended up at the principal's office. All the students accused Frank of attacking them. Frank was confused and upset. He could not make sense out of what they were saying and did not know what to say. The principal concluded that he must be guilty and suspended him from school for two days!

It was not until the next day that his mother called and said he had been able to tell her what had happened. In a quiet visit with the principal, Frank was able to explain what had happened. The principal believed him and apologized for what had

47

> *happened. It was a dramatic demonstration to me of the disabling aspect of listening confusion.*

This incident underscores the tremendous effect of stress on auditory processing. The confusion in understanding what was being said in this incident was indicative of Frank's listening confusion. The children were not making sense to Frank because their verbal descriptions were not consistent with what he was experiencing. He could not understand what was happening. When he could not make sense of what he heard, he did not know how to respond.

Our learners continually have the impact that listening confusion creates for them. It is often imbedded in other learning issues. Most of our learners have shared the frustration and panic that they have experienced when they did not understand what they were hearing. One of the primary coping mechanisms that they developed in attempting to relieve the frustration, was to dominate conversation situations. Four of the seven learners found this to be their most effective strategy.

It was very difficult to get a word in to a conversation with Tim. He controlled the conversation from the moment he walked in until he left. In one session I stopped attempting to redirect him and just sat and watched the clock behind him. He talked consistently for an hour. When I remarked about the time, he was startled to find that we had little time left for our therapy. He was unaware of time passing while he was talking.

Both Tim and Ron shared that they became aware of their difficulty in processing in elementary school. They felt at the time that it was complicated by distracting visual imagery. Tim found that he got many visual images and that he would be distracted by them. Ron shared an almost identical feeling. He felt that he was day dreaming with his visual images and it was keeping him from concentrating on what was being said.

The phenomenal experience that each of them repeated was that they decided to *shut off their visualizations* and only work with their listening. What they had identified as the problem was actually their attribute of greater strength. They shut down, consciously, their strength in learning because it distracted them in listening. One recalled making that decision in seventh grade and *"living in a world of words."* The other did it much earlier in second or third grade.

It is startling to think that children have the ability to recognize and make decisions in learning of this nature. They also experience the impact of their choices as life-long learning frustrations. Ron provided an excellent example of his confusion in recall, as he reported an incident which

49

happened when he was a high school student working in his father's tire and automotive business.

> *Ron - One of the things I remember in relation to my problems was obvious when I worked for my father in his business. I would have to make these deliveries and he would give me directions.*

> *JS - What kind of business did you have?*

> *R - Tires and automotive business, retail. So I would have to drive from our city to another in this big truck and pick up tires and drop tires off or pick up parts for repairing autos. He would give me these directions on how to find the place. After several failures at this sort of thing, I remember he said "now look at me in the eye" which was just the wrong thing to do, and he would say" now you are going to do this and you are going to go here."*

> *He would speak very slowly, as though I didn't even speak English, as though I was a foreigner. Then I would have to repeat them back to him. My mind was completely blank which is the way it is. I recall there was a certain amount of embarrassment going on and, with youth, impatience. So I would say "Dad, I got it. I can do it."*

50

So I'd get on the road and about ten minutes later, I'd say to myself, "Well, I've got to call at the first stop, I've got to call and figure out where I am!" Of course, I was lost as usual.

Ron illustrates the efforts of an intelligent learner to appear to be listening. Our learners developed a skill in appearing to be attending to what someone was saying. Actually, although they looked attentive they were verbalizing with their inner voice thoughts like. "Oh, no, I don't know what she is talking about," or "This is so boring, I will never be able to get it," Ron shared.

Ron - When people talk, I pretend to listen to what they are saying, but I really don't.

JS - I can see it on your face when you stop listening.

R - You can.

JS - You have a look of...I've got to interrupt... and I know you have left listening then.

R - Why do you think that is?

JS - You could probably answer this better than I, but I suspect it is an attempt to hold what you are thinking and to respond to it before you forget what you wanted to say. Does that register with you?

R - If you are spontaneous like I am, that is exactly right. If I can't compartmentalize information, which is a word I like to use, then I have to be immediate. It's that inability, or lack of confidence, to being able to hold information. Exactly. You are right.

JS - That is the impression I get from listening to you, and others, who experience that frustration and fear. It is very difficult to try to wait for someone to finish talking when you have something you want to say. I know that you are afraid that you will forget what you wanted to say. That has been your experience and that fear is very powerful.

Some of our learners are less tactful in controlling their need to interrupt or insert their thoughts in the conversation. This is an important indicator of the frustration that they experience. They are convinced that if they wait for a pause by the speaker, they will no longer be able to comment intelligently. They will *forget* what they wanted to say.

Children who blurt out answers or interrupt or dominate conversations often experience this listening inefficiency. It is a clear indicator that they are feeling a discomfort with the traditional flow of conversation. Each of our learners was aware that they were frequently accused of interrupting as children. They tended to develop a skill in making amusing remarks to distract the speakers. This was socially acceptable as an interruption and was often enjoyed by others. They became known for their wit or humor. In fact, it was a conscious effort to cover for fear and confusion.

Our learners have experienced reaching a point in listening which is best described as the *threshold of confusion*. We all experience this at different times. A secretary in an office experiences it, when four different bosses each hand him or her letters that must be completed within the next hour, and the telephone keeps ringing.

The feeling of urgency, panic and "What shall I do?"tilts the intellect into emotional confusion. The cat with three mice running around all at once gives us a good visual of the feeling. It is basically a logical response to extreme sensory overload. The cat does not know which mouse to chase first and often loses all of them in its indecision.

Our listeners experience the threshold of confusion when they experience auditory overload. All of a sudden the information ceases to be making sense to them, and they cannot process any more information. Since these learners experience frustration so frequently, they trigger the threshold of confusion at an earlier point than learners with greater confidence. Once a learner can recognize that they are approaching the threshold, they can choose to take control. They no longer have to continue crossing into it and experience *panic and frustration.*

> *Ron - All of these characters are starting to float on me. I can't make sense of what I am supposed to do.*

> *J - Take a breath and tell yourself that you can choose to take back the control. You may want to tell yourself that you want to clarify the instruction so that it will make sense again.*

> *R - You were wise not to respond to all the comments I first made when I came here. I felt there was something wrong with me, but now I am seeing that there isn't something wrong but it's an access thing. I hate that word. It's not using what I have.*

> *JS - Dang brain is sitting there and you haven't chosen to put it to work.*

> *R - It hasn't been used. My mind wants to say, "Well, why not?" Do you know how many people have said that to me? I get them so frustrated by asking so many questions so I can understand what they say.*

JS - It goes back to our premise we talked about a few times ago. When you hit the threshold of confusion, you instantly abandoned the ship. Now you are beginning to confront it. You are not going overboard so easily!

When I think of the threshold of confusion I always remember a good friend of mine. She is an extremely confident and powerful person. When we were flying back from a consulting trip, she was busy working on a project and totally in charge. All of a sudden the airplane hit some turbulence. She immediately dumped all her papers and books into the laps of the passengers on each side of her and grabbed onto the armrests with a look of total panic on her face. When the plane calmed down she reclaimed her materials and went back to work. In essence that is what I see you doing whenever you encounter the slightest bump.

R - Bump, that is a good analogy. It also puts it into perspective.

When we hit our threshold of confusion, we tend to forget all of the reasonable resources we have to respond to a situation. We toss out all the options and embrace panic as the solution.

In order to resolve this response pattern, we need to identify when we are starting to reach the confusion point. The earlier we can identify our direction, the more likely we are to be able to alter our course. For some learners it is an intellectual or verbal message.... "I'm starting to lose this." or "It's really hard to listen to him talking." For other learners it is emotional...an increase in heart rate, a feeling in the stomach, a need to shake her head - as though that would clear it. Whatever the sign, it will serve as a message that we need to take control of our listening and start to use one of our solutions.

One learner shared with me that he could not speak or write well. He wanted to be able to stand up and speak to groups of people with confidence. He felt that he could stand up and entertain with smart remarks but he could not communicate the information that was needed for his business purposes. The whole time he was standing up talking, his inner voice was pointing out who was not listening, that they seemed bored, and that he kept saying "and". He had a running critique going in his head.

It was helpful for him to understand, that our inner voice is a very powerful force in how successful we are with any task. Our inner voice has two levels: the *Critic Voice* and the *Guide Voice*. The basic, emotional level is the one that we call the Critic Voice. This is the one that points out everything we do or might do to make ourselves feel inadequate, foolish and stupid. We often have full tapes that the Critic Voice can plug in and get immediate results of feeling stupid. These are usually leftovers from things we have heard from significant people in our lives; mother tapes, teacher tapes, etc.

> I can't sing. [*Mother tape..."You can't carry a tune in a bucket."*]

> I am a terrible skier. [*Ski instructor tape.... "You look like a sick cow when you ski like that."*]

> I can't express my thoughts effectively. [*Father tape..."Think before you speak, what is the matter with you anyway?"*]

Over the years we begin to accumulate many of these Critic tapes associated with certain situations and feelings. We begin to *generalize* these messages and *associate* them with other situations. Now we not only cannot sing but we cannot play the piano!

We commonly use both of our inner voice resources in processing information. The Critic provides us with commentary and the *Guide Voice* dialogue provides us with information. The Guide Voice is much more supportive. It is respectful, caring, and oriented toward *solution* instead of criticism. It is this guiding voice, that we find supportive and helpful in being effective learners. It is the Guide Voice we need to begin using as the inner-voice, for accomplishing our goals.

It is helpful to image these as separate areas in our resourceful brain. **Our ears can only listen to and make sense of one voice at a time.** When we listen to the criticism - "You'll never get this." "You didn't get it right last time, how do you expect to do it this time?" "It's not making sense to you, you might as well give up." "She is going to think you are stupid." - we are unsuccessful. We find ourselves blocking the task we are attempting to do.

If we can *turn **off** the Critic Voice* and *turn **on** the Guide Voice* we can begin to find the solution, the answer, and engage in the process for accomplishing our intent. The Guide is likely to tell us "This is just a step along the way. We will get there eventually." "First we should begin by finding all of the information we need to resolve this." The Guide is solution- oriented.

> *Mark - I just panic when I start to think about memorizing all these pictures and names.*
>
> *JS - What are you saying to yourself? Let me hear your inner language [voice].*

58

M - I can't do this. There are too many and I've never done this many before. It's not fair.

JS - Wow, I felt like I was in your head listening with you. Thank you for letting me do that. Let's change the station on your inner radio. First, let's make a list of guiding statements versus critical statements. O.K.?

M - I have a hunch where this is going.

JS - Good hunch! Tell me Guide or Critic voice when I give you a statement.

We verbalized as many statements as we could think of and developed a list of statements. Then we identified which were criticisms and which were helpful - guide statements.

> *I can't do it.*
> *I never could figure this out.*
> *Last time I missed all of these and I am no better this time.*
> *I could figure it out if I listed all the variables.*
> *I have plenty of time to complete this task.*
> *I can pretend to do it and then not come back.*
> *I know I can do this if I ask the right questions.*

This process provided a distinct delineation of the difference between Critic and Guide voices that we use to give ourselves information. The next step was to begin to *shut down* the Critic voice.

> *JS - This time let's do the task again. Whenever you start to hear a Critic voice, you will want to tell it to "Shut up!". You can say NO or STOP IT or whatever you like. As soon as you have stopped it, you will follow it with a Guide statement like... "I can figure this out. I have plenty of resources to use."*
>
> *M - Okay, do I do it so you can hear?*
>
> *JS - It would be helpful to me but you can choose what is most comfortable.*
>
> *M - Okay, I am going to do these ten memory things and remember them till the end of the hour. That is what you want? [Nod] I am looking at the first one, but no association is coming to me. STOP. I started to hear myself say my memory couldn't do this. So instead I will say...its going to take me a while but I can do it.*
>
> *JS - Yes! You are using your inner guide voice. How are you feeling?*

M - Like I want to giggle. It strikes me as funny, talking to myself like this.

JS - We all hear ourselves talk all the time. Does it feel better than the feeling of panicking we had before?

M - Got that right!

Individuals who experience comprehension problems in their reading are experiencing these issues. They usually have some inefficiencies in their listening comprehension. *When we read we are listening to our inner voice.* This is the same as listening to someone speak.

Along with inefficiencies in auditory processing they have developed confusion with auditory conceptualization. In other words, when they read, the words do not communicate information, the information does not integrate and usually, the images that words can evoke, are missing.

Auditory conceptualization requires the combination of the attributes of auditory memory and visual imagery. We must be able to take in information and register it with both language and imagery. This skill requires adequate strength in each of these attributes.

Learning Victories

In order to establish auditory conceptualization we have found the *Auditory Conceptualization Using Stories* described in the Edu-Therapeutics Section to be very effective. Since it does not require *direct confrontation* of concept development it can be successful without being stressful. The need for reducing as much of the stress, panic and fear associated with learning, is an important consideration in the selection of therapeutic interventions.

Our learners benefit from gaining control over their inner voice, learning to listen to a solution-oriented inner language, and improving in their auditory memory skills. These interventions are successful and beneficial. There are a variety of characteristics that inter-relate in this process, and it is important to look at our processing speed and attention focus skills, which may impact on auditory development.

Chapter Six

HYPER-PROCESSING VS. DELAYED RESPONSE TIME

Everyone knows that if you are fast and finish first, you are the best!

Lucy looked at me like I was an idiot, when I told her that being fast and finishing first only counted in horse races! She informed me in her most exasperated voice... *"Everyone knows that you are the best if you finish first in class!"*

Of course, this was Lucy's observation in the classroom. It was probably the majority of the class's opinion, too. As students, we are taught to finish as quickly as possible. Our educational system prizes speed.

Lucy learned to finish first in the class. Since she could not read or spell in third grade, she would copy words from the page and fill in the blanks with those words and then proudly walk up to the teacher's desk and put the paper in the box. The other students were appropriately impressed with Lucy's speed.

The irritation Lucy was experiencing with my observations was closely associated with the anger she felt toward herself.

In fact, Lucy had a delay in her response time. She could not think of the correct answer and respond quickly. She wanted desperately to appear as though she were competent. She wanted most of all to <u>be</u> competent.

Lucy is a very bright individual. We know that from the scores we saw on her intelligence testing. Then why did she experience such frustration in learning to read, and why do intelligent learners have difficulty in reading? In some cases it is related to the response-time delay.

This energetic, spontaneous, witty young lady experienced a delay in her reaction time. Response time is one of the variables which is measured by the Test of Variables of Attention (TOVA) [Lawrence M. Greenberg, M.D., Department of Psychiatry, University of Minnesota, MN., reference in Appendix.] It is an excellent resource for identifying attention challenges.

The TOVA is a continuous-response task. The subject watches a computer screen and responds to targets which appear in the upper half of a box, and ignores targets which appear in the lower portion of the box. The task continues for twenty-two minutes. During the first portion of the task, there are more nontargets appearing than targets. The response-pacing requirement is relatively slow, and patience and concentration are important elements for success.

During the second portion of the task, there are many more targets than nontargets. This requires the subject to respond quickly and be able to discriminate, and maintain control of impulsivity, simultaneously. It measures four variables of attention:

Inattention: Identified when the subject fails to respond to a target. A learner with inattention is often accused of daydreaming in the classroom or being vague in response to surrounding stimuli. The learner does not appear to have adequate arousal to stimuli in the environment. Actual focus may be occupied with internal stimuli (thoughts) or focus on a different stimulus.

Impulsivity: Readily apparent because of the subject's active response to stimuli. The learner often responds to all stimuli. This includes stimuli which would appear to have low interest, anticipated stimuli which are not present yet, or a combination of stimuli. The learner will respond in anticipation of the target or will respond to nontargets during the assessment. She will have a particularly difficult time during the second half of the test when rapid discrimination between targets and nontargets is required.

Response Time: Reaction time inefficiencies are probably the most challenging of the attention-related issues. The time delay is not obvious to the observer because the time differentiation is measured in milliseconds. As teachers and parents we are unaware of this problem because we cannot see it. There are a variety of characteristics associated with this variable in attention. It is the primary issue in the majority of the learners who have shared in this presentation.

Variability: Inconsistency in response times is measured in this variable. A learner with challenges in this area, will demonstrate speeded responses and then slowed responses. The variation creates difficulty in responding efficiently.

A TOVA profile for a learner without attention issues shows standard scores which are similar to the individual's intelligence scores. *An average learner would be expected to have scores within a normal standard score range of 85-115. A bright learner would usually have higher scores, possibly between 110-130.*

Test of Variables of Attention	
Name: Sample	
Medication: No	
Omissions	103
Commissions	99
Response Time	97.5
Variability	102

Subjects who experience challenges with a variable will have scores which are below average (lower than 85) or which are significantly deviant (low) in comparison to their intellectual level.

Learners who experience challenges with attention, will usually find one or more of the variables to be significantly deviant on the TOVA. When this is an issue, it is important to address the attention variance.

Students who are attempting to learn to read and have a delay in their response time will experience serious reading delays. The timing that they experience in responding to a stimulus, will be the same whether it is a target on the screen, or a symbol or word on a page. It takes them longer to make the connection between the letter and sound than we would naturally expect.

We find that our "good" teachers continually *interrupt* these students while they are attempting to sound out a word. Instead of allowing the additional processing time, teachers feel compelled to assist in providing a prompt to the student to speed up their decoding. This *prompt* has the effect of re-starting the processing clock.

If a student is staring at the word <u>bat</u>, the teacher will often prompt by saying, "Sound it out, use your sounds." This intervention restarts the processing time. Before the student can continue into this effort, the teacher invariably prompts again with "Buh", the first sound is buh. This process continues with the prompts restarting the processing clock, until the word has been sounded out to the teacher's satisfaction, often, by the teacher!

Learners who experience this type of challenge in their processing time, have great difficulties in the classroom. They need considerable time even in one-to-one instruction before skills become automatic.

Even when the learner has succeeded in developing a reading system, this processing-time issue will continue to create frustration for them. Response time is critical in the processing of language. Learners with delays in response time, experience difficulty in listening for information. Young children appear to be not listening or ignoring instructions. They often make mistakes after just having been "told" how something is to be done. The delay in response time makes it difficult for them to integrate instructions in a timely, efficient manner. Processing multiple stimuli simultaneously is exceptionally confusing.

Adult learners with response-time issues often experience discouragement and depression. They continually feel out of synchrony with their skills and the performance. Ron was

68

very open in sharing his frustration with his response issues. He had great difficulty in finishing projects, classes and his own goals. He found that nothing sustained his interest for very long and he could not decide on a career direction. He reported that he could not listen very effectively because he could not remember what was being said. He consequently had numerous comprehension difficulties which extended into reading as well as into the processing of conversations.

The first profile shows the difficulty he was experiencing with attention. It is obvious that his Reaction Time is significantly delayed and Variability slightly elevated.

Test of Variables of Attention
Name: Ron
Medication: None

Omissions	100
Commissions	117
Response Time	**< 25 [T-108.8]**
Variability	**61**

Ron chose to work with his physician to assist in improving his attention. He was placed on a common attention medication. The TOVA was re-administered to help understand the effect of the medication on his performance. It is apparent that his Reaction Time actually worsened although his variability improved slightly.

```
┌─────────────────────────────────────────────────┐
│            Test of Variables of Attention        │
│         Name: Ron                                │
│         Medication: 20Mg. Ritalin, Generic       │
│                                                  │
│         Omissions              100               │
│         Commissions            122               │
│         Response Time          <25 [T-110]       │
│         Variability             80               │
└─────────────────────────────────────────────────┘
```

It is not unusual to see Reaction Time become even more delayed with certain medications. In fact, the most appropriate response is usually seen with either a significantly reduced dose of medication or a modification of diet. Two of the dietary elements which appear to stress response time in learners are dairy and sugar.

Ron felt that his medication intervention was helpful to him even though it did not relieve the difficulty with his response time. The addition of the medication actually nudged the T-score upward. [These T-scores are reported in a reverse order. An average is 50 but the lower scores indicate positive performance and higher scores indicate difficulty.] When Ron's physician reduced the amount of medication and Ron participated in an experiment of restricting his diet, his profile was consistently in the normal range.

Test of Variables of Attention

Name: Ron
Medication: 5Mg. Ritalin, Generic
Diet Restrictions: No dairy or sugar

Omissions	103
Commissions	99
Response Time	97
Variability	102

Ron later identified that there were other foods to which he showed a reaction. When he chose to restrict his diet, he was remarkably clear in his thinking and relaxed in his verbalizations. His impulsivity in interrupting, changing the subject, and controlling a conversation, was reduced. He appeared to be at peace in his communication.

Teachers and others who observed Lucy *in action* would have identified that she was *impulsive.* She blurted out information, she could concentrate for a few seconds before interrupting herself, and she constantly talked about whatever she was thinking. She found most tasks terribly "boring" and was very difficult to keep on task, even in a one-to-one situation.

71

She had been recommended for medication and had taken ritalin for a number of months. She hated taking the medication and consistently reported that it made her *feel funny*. Her family felt that it seemed to dull her and that she was not "fun and spirited". Even her pediatrician agreed that it radically changed her personality.

When we observed a TOVA for Lucy it became clear why she disliked the ritalin so much. She actually did not have an impulsive disorder. She was having great difficulty in processing external stimuli and in her response time.

Test of Variables of Attention	
Name: Lucy	
Medication: None	
Omissions	< 25
Commissions	77
Reaction Time	46
Variability	< 25

Once we understood what Lucy was experiencing in her response time, and skill in responding to stimuli in her environment, it became obvious why she was miserable on the medication. It would have made her response time and ability to respond even slower!

The impulsivity which was observed with Lucy was really her attempt to respond quickly. Since she could not record the information as quickly as she needed it, she would verbalize about anything until she could make sense of the information.

One day we were working on her addition facts and I asked, "Two plus what makes ten?" Lucy responded immediately, "Red, blue, purple and.....*eight.*" I must have been looking at her somewhat stunned because she continued with.."Two plus eight makes ten. That's what I said, eight. What's wrong with you?"

We suggested that Lucy and her family work with her nutrition in order to improve her processing efficiency. During one session she was having her typical difficulty with remaining on task. We were working on the spelling words which she had been assigned for the week in her classroom. This was Thursday and her test was the next day. After she studied the words for forty-five minutes and the *right* interventions and techniques were employed, I decided to check on her progress. A copy of her paper follows on the next page.

As a fifth grader, Lucy could not even number the paper consecutively. She was rotating symbols [b/d] and sequences of sounds. She could barely construct the letter symbols. Some of the letters she wrote were incomplete [note second P in Mississippi and last letter in Florida in circle]. She

73

could not maintain the numbering system in setting up her paper. Not only did she repeat the numeral 10 twice but she followed the numeral 19 with 12. When I nudged her to point out her error. She angrily wrote in the 20 but did not correct her error.

When I asked her to tell me what she had eaten that day, she reported that her breakfast had been French toast with syrup, and that she had chocolate milk with her lunch. She could not stay on task at all and it was obvious that her learning was severely suffering. We were very discouraged with our ability to make consistent progress for Lucy. She was equally frustrated and had become an expert at avoiding work.

We requested that her family assist her in monitoring her diet prior to her next session. They were very cooperative and Lucy appeared for her lesson the following Thursday, dairy and sugar free.

Nov. 30. 1995
Spelling

French toast
Syrup
Choc milk

1 waner
2 turkey
3 Sugar
4 total
5 wonsel fuel
6 telephone
7 television sun
8 Holiday
9 November
10 street
10 cafidanu   alabama
12 Mississippi
13
14
15
16
17
18
19
12

20

Flora

Ao te

We began the lesson by dictating her words from the prior week without any intervening practice. Her organization was greatly improved. The page has the *feeling* of organization and clarity in contrast to the first page which is markedly chaotic. She had no difficulty with her numbering system. All of the symbols are more consistent in size and spacing. There was an absence of symbol rotations and good accuracy in letter formation. She had several single letter spelling errors which could be easily corrected. Her response is shown on the next page.

In the *Burden of Intellect* chapter we showed the comparative scores during two administrations of the Wechsler Intelligence Scale for Children -III. Although in November, 1995 Lucy was working with her diet and noting significant changes in her performance, by March she had returned to a typical diet. She was having particular difficulty at school. Her resource teacher gave her candy for working in her special program. In fact, for the triennial assessment with the resource teacher and school psychologist, the teacher gave her a jelly bean for each math problem she attempted. Her final score showed that she had regressed a full year and a half from the prior year in her math score.

The comparative score in her intellectual testing was based on a difference in her diet. When the March assessment was administered, Lucy was eating foods with no restrictions.

1 turkey

2 tennessee

3 alabama

4 floritda

5 November

6 total

7 Sugar

8 wire

9 Halliday

10 wonderful

11 straitght

12 telephone

13 television

14 Mississippi

15

16

17

18

19

20

12-14-95
No sugar.

77

Learning Victories

When the assessment was re-administered six months later she had been clear of her sensitive foods for a week prior to the assessment. A review of the assessment scores illustrates the difference in her organizational and performance skills with an adjusted diet.

Wechsler Intelligence Scale for Children - III		
	3/1/96	8/30/96
Verbal I.Q.	90	**106**
Performance I.Q.	98	**131**
Full Scale I.Q.	93	**120**

Lucy's processing time is significantly stressed by her consumption of dairy and sugar. She has been working specifically on monitoring her ingestion of these items. It is very difficult for both Lucy and her family. The more effective she is in her efforts, the more appropriate she is in learning.

These observations are not isolated case studies. We are identifying a distinct profile which appears to be associated with a slowing in response time and a reaction to dairy products and/or sugar or other foods. In some instances, just the elimination of dairy products enables the student to process in a more organized manner. Many of these learners had milk allergies as infants and often had chronic ear infections.

We are working on a consultive basis with a group of home schooling families on the East Coast. These parents have been impressive because of their commitment to identifying the issues their children are experiencing and their follow through in implementing solutions. Matthew is nine years old and has been home-schooled for the past year. His mother felt that he has both the Visual Symbol Confusion and Attention Focus Disruption types of dyslexic learning styles. [Reference:*You Don't Have to Be Dyslexic*, Joan M. Smith, SCI Distributors, 15608 S. New Century Dr., Gardena, CA.]

Matthew writes many letters backward. He has extreme difficulty in writing and frequently loses his place on the paper. He experiences the same confusion in reading. He often runs his letters together as he writes. When he was in school, he could not read fast enough to keep up with the class and was humiliated for not completing his work.

His mother was pleased because Matthew was happier being home schooled, but she was frustrated that she was not seeing him progress in learning. She reported that when he rode a bicycle, he tilted the bike to the left and his body and bike formed a V shape. When he picked up a toy, he would often hold something in one hand and then use the other hand to do something different. Sometimes he forgot what was in the other hand and dropped it.

79

Learning Victories

This is a sample of his handwriting at the time of his evaluation:

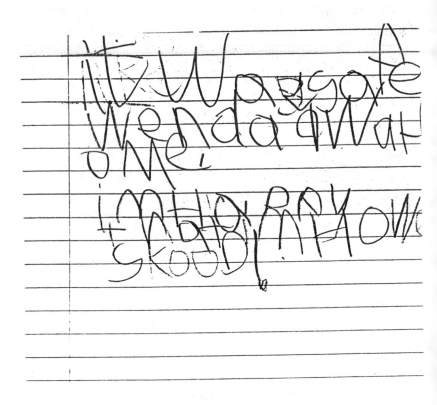

["It was safe when dad was home. I am happy I am home schooled.]

We were advised that he had a milk allergy and had chronic ear infections. He was drinking milk, however, and did not have a restricted diet. His mother was quite anxious to try a two-week experiment and remove dairy products and restrict sugar intake. This is a sample of Matthew's writing after two weeks of restricted diet. Radical changes are apparent in his organizational ability, size of the letters and letter formation.

Oct.23

light flashlight

ho use brickhouse

self myself

grand prize

Learning Victories

The difference in Matthew's writing was very apparent. He began to experience organization for the first time. His frequency of rotations of symbols diminished significantly. He still appeared to have difficulty with content and language orientation. Matthew's mother decided to maintain his diet with nutritional supplements to replace the dairy benefits. Within four months time, he was showing not only improved handwriting, but excellent organization, spacing and language skills. A sample of his writing illustrates these changes.

2/97

I want to learn to whistle.
I've always wanted to.
fix my mouth to do it but
The whistles won't come
Through

To call a dog

for fun

To be a bird

to make music

As startling as these changes appear to be, the important factor is that the organizational skills which are apparent, are indicative of greater changes. Matthew is ready for organizing and sequencing stimuli. He is now ready to develop a reading system and to respond to instruction. His mother is delighted with his processing changes, and finds that he is now learning at an appropriate pace.

We worked with a fifteen year-old-high school student named Rita. She was a highly-intelligent student who spent many hours every evening dedicated to her homework. Even with her extreme effort, she made average grades. She was very discouraged and frustrated with her learning; especially since her friends did not study as long as she did and yet they made far better grades.

Rita experienced subtle challenges in her spelling and word-attack skills. They were slightly below her age and grade level on standard tests. She was above a high school level on General Information and Comprehension skills.

In our efforts to better understand her learning style, we administered several subtests from a "dated" but sensitive assessment tool - The Detroit Test of Learning Aptitude. [The DTLA has been revised several times since the original version, however, the same three subtests are not all included in the revisions.] On these three tasks, Rita's challenges with processing were quite apparent. Her ability to repeat a series of unrelated words was limited to a five-unit level.

We worked with Rita for eighteen months, one hour each week, and her academic score improved to above-high-school level in every area. The exceptions to her progress were in her processing scores on the DTLA which did not change. Even with her improvement in academics, she was still frustrated and working long hours to accomplish her studies. The comparison of scores from her initial assessment and the repeated assessment appear below.

Detroit Test of Learning Aptitude Name: Rita		
	11/93	3/95
Auditory Attention for Unrelated Words	8-0	8-5
Visual Attention for Objects	11-8	11-3
Auditory Attention for Related Syllables (Sentences)	13-0	13-0

In April of 1995, we suggested that Rita have a TOVA, the results of which are shown next. It was apparent that the issue that was continuing to plague Rita, was a slowing in her response time.

```
Test of Variables of Attention
Name: Rita
Medication: None

Omissions          107
Commissions        114
Reaction Time      < 70
Variability         93
```

As a teenager, Rita was resistive to any restrictions in her diet. She did not want to take medication and was still having great difficulty in schoolwork. By mid-summer Rita had relaxed enough from the school year that she was willing to look ahead to next year. She chose to cooperate with an *experiment* with her diet. After two weeks on the diet, we re-administered the TOVA and her profile shows the dramatic difference.

```
Test of Variables of Attention
Name: Rita
Medication: None
Restricted Diet: No sugar or dairy

Omissions          107
Commissions        107
Reaction Time      109
Variability        113
```

85

Rita begrudgingly admitted that she felt more organized and could "think better". Her DTLA subtests were re-administered and showed that she was processing information with far greater comfort.

Detroit Test of Learning Aptitude	
Name: Rita	
Restricted Diet: No sugar or dairy	
	8/95
Auditory Attention for Unrelated Words	15-7
Visual Attention for Objects	18-3
Auditory Attention for Related Syllables	15-7

When Rita returned to school she chose to use her diet to improve her school grades. She began to excel in her studies and no longer needed tutorial intervention.

Tim, our bank manager, experienced challenges with his attention in processing information, and organizing his time management. His profile is different than those which showed a slowing of response time. Tim experienced challenges with his impulsivity. His profile showed the deviation of his impulsivity as it is measured in Commissions.

Test of Variables of Attention
Name: Tim
Medication: None

Omissions	90
Commissions	**36**
Response Time	109
Variability	85

Consistent with the typical characteristics of impulsivity, Tim wanted a *quick fix* for his attention challenge. He requested medication from his physician and was initially placed on 20 Mg. of ritalin. He found that he was unable to sleep. He became frightened because of a "pounding heart". His dosage was reduced to 5 Mg of ritalin. His second TOVA showed improvement in his impulsivity [Commissions.]

Test of Variables of Attention
Name: Tim
Medication: 5 Mg. Ritalin

Omissions	100
Commissions	**73**
Response Time	108
Variability	116

There was apparent improvement in Tim's impulsivity;

however, he continued to show that it was not resolved. At the same time he continued to experience spells of what he described as a "racing heart". He decided to abandon his medication intervention. He chose to work with the diet control for one week. This was exceptionally difficult for Tim because his family did not think it was important for him to work with his diet. He chose to persevere, and at the end of a week of eliminating sugar and dairy from his diet his TOVA profile reflected the change.

```
        Test of Variables of Attention
      Name:   Tim
      Medication: None
      Restricted Diet:   No dairy or sugar

      Omissions                 100
      Commissions               110
      Response Time             105
      Variability               115
```

Tim experienced good organizational skills and a calm, relaxed manner on his diet. He became very aware of the difference when he ingested restricted foods.

Several months after this assessment had been completed, Tim came in for our Wednesday session. He talked without stopping for twelve minutes. I had ceased to listen and was clocking him. Finally, I signaled him to cover his mouth and stop talking. He did so and looked at me with frantic eyes.

JS - What are you experiencing?

T - I can't stop talking. I have been talking for the past three days. It was my birthday on Saturday, and my family made ice cream and cake and lasagne as a special dinner for me. We had the left-overs the next two nights and its still in my system.

Tim explained that his body was "racing" and that he was having a difficult time working. We talked about the need for his diet restrictions, and the impact on his work and health, when he *loaded* himself with these particular foods. It was obviously difficult for him to control his eating, without the support of his family. They needed to realize that he required their cooperation.

These are individual case examples. We cannot generalize that everyone who experiences a delay in response time has a reaction to dairy products or sugar. The *impact on the processing and skills* demonstrated in these cases should lead us to consider the ***impact of what we eat on how we think.*** There is a connection for many people.

We have developed a checklist of typical characteristics of individuals who experience a delay in reaction time. When six to eight of these characteristics are observed consistently, it is appropriate to recommend that the learner be evaluated for response-time challenges.

Learners who experience the frustration of a delay in their processing, often engage in behaviors which confuse their teachers and family. They tend to have difficulty in listening and find learning boring. They will appear impulsive or hyperactive. In fact, these behaviors mask their perceived slowness in thinking. When the response-time issues are resolved, these learners can engage in organized behavior and systematic learning.

ATTENTION FOCUS
DELAYED REACTION TIME

Check the ☺ for behaviors which are observed frequently or consistently:

☺ 1. Frequently responds with "Huh?" when provided with information or asked a question.

☺ 2. Has poor listening skills or identified auditory memory difficulty.

☺ 3. Has great difficulty completing work assignments in class.

☺ 4. Appears to have more homework than other siblings or classmates because of speed of working.

☺ 5. Avoids doing work or appears to be "lazy".

☺ 6. Daydreams during class time.

☺ 7. Difficulty in recognizing words in reading.

☺ 8. Does not appear to improve despite extra or special help.

☺ 9. Responds with "uh, huh" as though the information is understood, but cannot follow through with task.

☺ 10. Seems to have a delay in responding to questions.

☺ 11. Appears to ignore or avoid listening to instructions.

☺ 12. Verbal responses to questions or conversations do not appear related to the topic.

☺ 13. Starts to respond with unrelated information and then switches to appropriate response.

☺ 14. Difficulty in comprehending reading.

☺ 15. Raises hand to respond to question but forgets answer when called upon.

☺ 16. Doing timed tasks/tests is very difficult.

☺ 17. Gets lost in copying materials or staying on task.

91

Chapter Seven

GETTING THE PICTURE:
VISUAL IMAGERY AS AN ATTRIBUTE

When I think of myself, I could use the analogy of a television. A television has audio and visual and the mind does too. If you press the mute button you obviously just get the picture. If the picture tube is screwed-up you just get the audio.

Well, if this fits people like me, I have a very poor picture tube and I'm not getting a very good picture!

Imagery, picturing, visualization, or whatever we want to label it, is an important attribute in learning. It is the ability to generate an image in our mind. The image may be of something which we have seen before, or it may be something creative and newly-constructed. One person's image is likely to be very different from that of another person's.

It is important to understand that our learners experienced two misconceptions about visual imagery. First, they usually believed that <u>other people</u> could visualize so clearly that the image appeared to be real. Second, they felt that their ability to visualize information was inferior to others.

Since we cannot experience someone else's image, we really have no way of knowing how clear and precise their picture appears. In our study and analysis of imagery, one important reality has emerged. Most people experience images which are vague and without great detail. An image is wispy and vague around the edges, especially when we keep our eyes open. It is usually not as vivid as a dream; but if we concentrate on creating details with our image, it can become complex. We have to *concentrate* on the image in order to embellish it.

There are several types of imagery with which we can experiment in our learning. The first is *concrete visualizations.* This is the imaging of something we have actually seen. For instance, we can look at a spelling word on a page [bread] and then look up and image it on a wall. We may see an image of the letters and be able to point to them and spell the word. We actually have seen that particular image including the order of the letters and the type of lettering.

Next we can manipulate that concrete image if we choose. For instance, we can image the last letter being moved to the beginning of the word. Then our image would look more like [dbrea]. We have creatively altered our concrete image. We call this a *constructive* visual memory or image. We are manipulating the visual information from a concrete image into something different.

In contrast to concrete images, we have *creative* images. These are the images which may come from language input (reading, listening or thinking) or from playing with visual elements creatively. These are not necessarily images that we have already seen or that we recall seeing.

We use creative imagery when we read a novel about Andalusia and the village is described to us as *...it appeared that the village consisted of a conglomeration of mud blocks, placed in an orderly fashion over the side of the hill, with narrow passages between the blocks to serve as streets and accommodate the mule carts of the merchants.*

Although we may never have seen a picture of Andalusia or a village of this type, the words create an image for us. We can build upon this image as details are added for us. *The desert sun baked the mud structures each day until they had become the color of a ripe persimmon and blended with the surrounding earth.* Now we can add color to our picture and expand on the details as we read.

We can image our own details because of some past experience or something we have heard or seen. We bring this information to our image and embellish it. Individuals

94

who enjoy reading, often report that a story *plays before them*. They mean they are enjoying the imagery which the author has created with his or her words.

In order to be effective learners we need to develop several skills to support our visual attribute. We require an adequate visual memory, visual discrimination skill, and awareness that we are able to image as a learning strategy.

Visual Memory - This skill enables us to recall a visual image and the component parts of something we have seen. By the time we are eight years old we should be able to recall six units or items from visual memory. We continue to refine this skill as we mature, however, seven units of information is consistently an adequate memory span for most adults.

Visual Discrimination - Skill in discriminating between images involves both memory and analysis. If we look at the word *form* and then compare it to the word *from* we will notice that there are both similarities and differences in the images. The individual letter units are the same but the order is different. For many learners these words appear to be the same and are easily confused. This is an important skill for reading efficiency.

Visual Imagery as a Strategy - The use of imagery is a primary strategy in learning. We need to recognize its

95

utility in acquiring information and being productive. Visual imagery can be useful in developing an outline for a paper, in organizing information, in relating to a schedule, and in most of the tasks we are asked to do both as children and adults.

A common observation from several of our learners was that they had found that their visual attributes had been so confusing to them as youngsters that they had *shut them off.* This was startling information when we first heard it. The idea that a child could decide to turn off a major learning channel, or would even identify it as interference, was difficult to understand. By now this has been reported so frequently during our sessions with different learners, that there is no doubt that it does happen and is an issue. Mark shared his experience in a session.

> *Mark - As a kid I used to do these visually, but I thought things were wrong with me and I stopped them. I thought everyone else was doing it with their language so I did it too.*

> *JS - I recall your comment about how distracting your visualizations were. But I am pleased that you recall using your visual system, it speaks to the fact that it is still available to you and intact!*

M -What if I can't remember what you are saying to me? How can my visual system make a difference?

JS - We are going to learn about your visual system by activating it for you. We will use these Mind Benders *as an activity to experiment with it. I have a word I use, but I am not certain it is a real word... it is concretize.*

M - I like it, I know what it means.

JS - Yes, it does communicate. We want to make the visual image <u>concrete</u> *so I say I want to concretize it! Anyway, the idea is we want it in a concrete and solid form. If it is in concrete it will be really hard to lose.*

M - You know, I think those numbers I put on that shelf are kind of like that. [He imaged three numerals on the book shelf during his previous lesson. He doubted that he would recall them because he did not believe that he had a working visual memory.] *I am not even thinking about it and the numbers are still sitting up there. You have no idea how this delights me. It is really my mind working!*

Mark was experiencing his visual memory working for the first time that he could acknowledge. He had chosen to ignore his visualization skill because of the confusion he thought it created for him in learning as a youngster. Now he understood that he needed to reactivate it. He could achieve his goals more effectively if he utilized all of his *brain resources* efficiently.

Many of our learners experience challenges in visualization because they have not stretched their visual memory skills. Sometimes they have a digit recall of four units of information. Obviously a four-letter recall does not support reading conveniently. This is a classic *Visual Symbol Confusion* type of dyslexic learning style. It makes it difficult for the learner to develop a reading system. They do not easily recall sight-words and often confuse what they are seeing.

Nancy, our nationally ranked athlete, experienced a form of this visual memory confusion. Her experiences in school mirror that of many of our clients.

Susan Smith - Nancy, how did your specific learning style impact on your school efforts and your work?

Nancy - I always described my learning style as, I read what I think I see, rather than what I see. So a lot of times I don't have the perception of it correctly. When it comes to directions and things like that I am really stuck. I won't be certain of what I am reading and I get stuck between what it says and what I think it says and I usually miss something. If someone were to just verbalize it, I would understand right away.

It can be really frustrating because I will be reading along and I see key words jump out at me whether it be at the end of the sentence or the middle . Then I have to go back and decipher what that whole message is and figure it out from beginning to end. A lot of time I will just take the key words and guess at the meaning of what it is trying to say .

The worst time is when they pass out a sheet and say read this and we are going to discuss it in class.

SS - What kind of response do you have to that?

N - It's like a panic attack because I am still reading along and everyone else is sitting there twiddling their thumbs and saying "Let's get on with it". And the more time pressure there is, the more I have no idea what it is about, even though I may have read the first three paragraphs while everyone else was going along comfortably at speed. Knowing it is in a timed situation, switches on this gear of stress.

It's the same with reading aloud. If there is a pressure to read in class, I won't see what is on the page. Even if it were my own writing and I knew what it said, I wouldn't be able to do it. It would be a panic, can't breathe kind of situation. I think it stems from the pressure at an early age to do it.

SS- Do you recall experiencing this a small child?

N - No, I can remember times in high school. That is such a vulnerable age anyway. I can still picture those classes. Once in English and once in journalism class. The teacher said... "I know you have dyslexia but stand up and read anyway, it doesn't matter. I don't care what the records say, you are full of baloney."

SS - Do the words blur or move?

N - It's kind of like they are shut-off. It's not necessarily a blank page, but the words might as well be written in Chinese. They don't make any sense.

My writing and spelling can be somewhat the same. I know what I am saying and I leave the letters off the end of the words. Other times I put all the letters in the words but I am putting them in the wrong order.

100

> *Even when I go back over and read it, I am seeing it*
> *the way I wrote it and it looks fine. It will be in the*
> *right order in my mind because all the right letters*
> *are in there. Like with **come**, I leave the e off or*
> *sometimes I write **ome** and leave the c off. Most of*
> *the time now I can go back and catch it. I am looking*
> *forward to a little bit more, too.*

Nancy found that the school system did not know how to teach the way she needed to learn. Her instructors did not recognize her powerful learning attributes. She was placed in remedial classes in grade school.

> *N - When I was in grade school they were pulling us*
> *out of school and taking us over to the remedial*
> *classes. They would do repetitive stuff over and over.*
> *I would say...”Wait a minute, I don't belong in this*
> *grade. ”*

Nancy is very bright and articulate. In school she tended to ignore her visual confusion and learn through her powerful listening system. Since her dyslexic learning style was visually obvious in her writing and reading, her instructors and counselors did not know how to assist her in using her talents.

> *N -All through school I could memorize information*

101

easily. In high school everything was so remedial, so easy. I couldn't understand why the other kids couldn't get it. I just memorized what the teacher said and I'd say, "Come on guys, its not so hard." It made so much sense to me. I would just feel like, "Okay, I got it. Let's move on."

In high school the instructors would say, "Oh, no, Nancy, you can't do that because..." They would always try to hold me back. I would have to say, "Let me show you, you don't have a clue. I'm better than that. I can get through."

My counselors in high school kept saying, "Don't even apply to a college, you will never get through. Don't get a P.E. major, it will be too hard. You can't take a second language." They would always talk me down. They were supposed to be pointing in the right direction in life. They are one of the reasons I went to Europe. I always wanted to learn a second language. I went to school in Austria. I hooked up with an au pair system and bought myself my own one-way ticket to Europe, got into school and learned German in less than a year. I learned it incredibly fast. It was exciting.

There is a strong tendency in our schools to look at one of a learner's attributes and assume that all of the other attributes are at the same level. This is true when the attribute viewed is intelligence... "You are bright. You can do it, if you will try." Or when it is visual confusion, which is very obvious and easy to see... "You won't be able to do that, do something easier." In fact, all of our attributes are likely to be at different levels of competence. That is what makes us unique as learners and establishes our different interests.

Visual memory skills can be developed and extended to be useful in learning and performing concrete recall, constructive image development and creative imagery. Learners benefit from learning to use their visualization skills and to developing constructive visualizations as a strategy for increased retention.

Mark did an exercise in constructive visualization. The task required him to create an image associated with a sentence in order to anchor the key information or facts. The exercise used a selection about John Kennedy. The task was for Mark to anchor the information by creating a picture. This is a marvelous visualization exercise and is discussed in detail in the *Edu-Therapeutics Section, Story Imaging Technique.*

> *JS - On that door we are going to image a frame for a picture. Can you see the frame?*

Mark - Yes, I am putting it in the top half of the door.

JS - The statement is..John F. Kennedy was born in 1917. What type of image would you like to put in the frame that will help you remember that information?

M - I see a New Years Eve type baby with a sash on and the sash has 1917 written on it and JFK.

JS - The next statement says... John was the second of nine kids. Place your frame and then describe your image.

M - I will put it on the bottom half of the door. Can I make them a baseball team? [Nod] I have them all lined up and he is the second tallest.

JS - Just to review, what is in the frame on top?

M - A baby with a sash with a date 1917 and initials.

JS - And here? [Pointing to the lower part of he door.]

M - The Kennedy baseball team and he is the second tallest so we know he was the second oldest.

104

JS -He grew up in Boston, how can we include that?

M - They have on red socks - the Boston Redsocks.

JS - His father was a business man and both his grandfathers were in politics.

M - Stop, I see his father in a three-piece suit. It is so clear. I can see him standing there and he has a watch in his hand, a pocket watch. I do see it.! The grandfathers are standing right behind him.

JS - What is over there? (Pointing to second frame.)

M - The Kennedy baseball team with the Boston socks and he is the second oldest. And in the next frame, there is the father, who is a business man and the two grandfathers that were in politics. This is great, it is working. And I didn't think I had a memory!

JS - These are picture memories and they won't go away.

M - But I start to panic and I think they will go away. Are you surprised that I am able to do this?

JS - No, I am not surprised. I believe that you will be

> *very successful doing this.*
>
> *M - I didn't know it. It's weird, its working.*
>
> *JS - We will leave the pictures on the wall for you to reference later if you wish. They will stay for you. When we do our relaxation today we will focus on the good visual skills and memory you have.*

This is an excellent technique for anchoring specific information for a purpose. For instance, a speaker may use it to anchor the main points of the speech. By just glancing at the imaged boxes the information will flow.

Since imagery is an important part of reading it is essential to activate imagery associated with words. There are a variety of techniques we use in Edu-Therapeutics to increase comprehension. Most of these techniques do not involve reading and imaging. It is more beneficial to establish the skill apart from reading. Then we can transition it easily and with little effort.

One of the challenges we usually experience is that the learner will have expectations for what they *should be* doing. For instance, when a learner is asked to relax and image information, there is often an expectation that they should recall *all the information.* It is critical to reduce these expectations and to refute them as soon as we are aware of their existence.

Melody - So, you are sure, I shouldn't expect to be automatic yet. I can keep going up levels in visual imagery and not expect to image everything or to hear everything.

JS - Absolutely, you are an imperfect person, along with the rest of us, so I guess you won't be able to hear everything. The operative word is everything! Maybe only every other thing!

M - Sometimes I seem to lose my concentration.

JS - Yes, it is wonderful how willful our brains can be. Here you are listening to information about the rain forest and they tell you how the rain is so heavy it pelts the leaves and knocks down the tender growth. And right in the middle of the information, you recall walking out of a restaurant in Acapulco and walking into a rain that was so heavy it was like walking in a waterfall.

This is a human thing to do. When you start dealing with constructive or creative imagery, it often will take you down side-streets.

> *M - I am catching up with the classics. I have "Pride and Prejudice" to read now.*
>
> *JS - That wasn't quite as frivolous as I would like for right now. I would like you to choose something really easy. It will allow you to do more with your visualization because it will not require so much energy. In fact, you might want to borrow some Agatha Christie from the library. You can take a quick trip to England with her by listening to a tape of one of her stories.*
>
> *And as you are listening if your mind starts to wander, its okay. Just relax and enjoy the experience. It is just for fun and part of our experiments.*
>
> *M - Yes, I remember, no expectations, just do it and enjoy it!*

Imagery is an important attribute for our learners to possess. It requires adequate memory and awareness that it is a skill which can be used. The exercises in Edu-Therapeutics provide adequate experience and opportunity to develop memory from increasing digit recall to visualization-strategy application.

Chapter Eight

EDU - THERAPEUTICS:
A Specialized Learning System

In Edu-Therapeutics the intent is to use what will work to resolve learning frustration and inefficiency. The focus begins on the attributes of learning which we require for effective and efficient learning. When our primary learning attributes are supportive, then we have the skills with which to learn.

The basic Edu-Therapeutic techniques were described in *"You Don't Have to Be Dyslexic"*. It described three unique types of dyslexic learning styles which create confusion and frustration for learners. The systems for resolving those learning styles are described in detail in both the first and second edition of the book.

In this presentation, the specific techniques used for the learners we have met through the preceding chapters will be shared. Many of these techniques have been developed after the previous publication and will provide new alternatives to resolving learning inefficiencies.

ASSESSMENT

Edu-Therapeutics uses a programming device which is called the ***Competency Assessment Battery (CAB)***. It is a series of computerized tasks which provide an observation of the learner in action. It measures memory in a new manner. Three types of memory tasks are utilized in the CAB for evaluating visual and auditory recall. The first is for immediate memory. For this task a series of symbols appear on the screen to be matched with the choices immediately below. This type of memory requires that the learner be able to discriminate the sequence of symbols. The auditory version of this task has the display of choices in front of the learner while he or she is hearing the stimulus series. The learner just chooses which of the series that he or she just heard.

The second type of memory involves short-term recall of the stimulus item. For instance, on the visual series, the learner sees a series of symbols, and then they disappear for five seconds. Then several variations of the symbols including the one which was displayed will appear. The learner must choose the correct series. During the auditory task, the learner hears the series, then waits five seconds for the choices
to appear on the screen, and he or she selects the correct series.

The third type of memory is unique. It requires a constructive memory task. A series of symbols are displayed for the learner. Then they disappear after five seconds and a selection of single symbols appear. The learner must reconstruct the series by selecting each of the symbols in order. For the auditory assessment, the learner hears the series of symbols to be selected, waits for the items to appear and then selects each of the symbols.

This third type of memory is closely related to spelling. Learners who have difficulty with this task often have great trouble in recalling the sequence of letter symbols required for a word.

Another observation of a learner's performance can give insights into his or her ability to maintain attention on task. When a profile on memory subtasks shows that the learner gets an easy one, then misses the next more difficult item, but then gets harder ones, we are often looking at an attention issue rather than a memory inefficiency. It is helpful, in establishing intervention strategies, to know what creates the underlying inefficiency.

There are thirty-two different subtasks on the CAB. They provide information about many of the learning attributes and the effectiveness in using these skills. The Melvin-Smith Learning Centers provide technical support and consultation for teachers and therapists as they are learning to interpret information and provide effective therapy with the CAB.

EDU-THERAPEUTICS - TRAINING TECHNIQUES

Edu-Therapeutics training system teaches that there are many techniques, systems and materials which are effective in resolving learning challenges. We advise using as many of the effective solutions for improving learning as possible. A truly effective therapist has many resources from which to choose for working with different learners. There is no single system which will work for every learner. Anyone, who believes that one system works for all, is ignoring brain research and the compatible understanding of attribute recognition. A reading guide is included to assist in accessing systems which may be beneficial for specific learner needs.

Edu-Therapeutics is built on a processing model. It is our belief that learning is sequential and that there are essential skills which must be learned in order to support complex learning tasks. The processing mode places the primary learning functions or skills first. Then we share the more complex processing which we describe as strategies, and finally the most complex processing, which is the actual integration of these skills enabling reading, writing, calculating and complex task performance. The phases of this learning model illustrate the skills in processing at each level. This is discussed and applied in detail in the training portion of *You Don't Have to Be Dyslexic.*

LEARNING ATTRIBUTES MODEL
ACTIVE PHASES OF LEARNING

PROCESSING SKILLS	STRATEGIES EXECUTIVE FUNCTION SKILL	ACADEMIC SKILLS

MEMORY SKILLS
  VISUAL
  AUDITORY
  MOTOR
 	
ATTENTION FOCUS
  TIME SENSE
  SCREENING
 	
MOTOR
COORDINATION
 	
LANGUAGE
	VISUALIZATION
	  VISUAL CONCEPT
	
	RE-VERBALIZATION
	  AUDITORY CONCEPT
	
	INTEGRATION OF
	SYSTEMS
	
	IDENTIFICATION OF
	STRATEGIES
	
	STUDY SKILLS
		READING
		  WORD ATTACK
		  COMPREHENSION
		
		SPELLING
		
		WRITTEN LANGUAGE
		
		NUMERIC
		CALCULATION AND
		REASONING
		
		SUBJECT CONTENT

Edu-Therapeutics evaluates each of these learning systems in an effort to understand the most basic level of inefficiency that the learner is experiencing. Most learners who are experiencing challenges in academic functioning actually have very basic inefficiencies in memory, attention or language functioning. In thirty years of using this system, and our work with over twelve thousand learners, we have consistently found that academic skills do not improve to an independent functioning level until the processing skills and strategy application have been developed.

It is because of our focus on resolving processing inefficiencies that we can create independent learners. Our emphasis is on building foundation skills, integrating strategies for applying the skills and transitioning these skills for academic and career application. There is no doubt that it is this sequence of learning steps that resolves learning disabilities.

The Edu-Therapeutic program interventions which follow have been effective in developing attribute strengths and skills. They include the following:

Edu-Therapeutic Techniques

Memory Grids - Association Memory Training
Auditory Conceptualization
Visual Conceptualization
Writing as a Visual-Verbal Process
Time and Space Conceptualization

These techniques may be adapted to a wide-range of age levels from elementary through adult years by adjusting the stimulus topics or materials employed.

MEMORY GRIDS
Association Memory Training

Memory Grids are one of the most effective and efficient resources to use for increasing memory, applying strategies for learning and improving confidence. The grids may be used for recalling information from multiplication tables to word definitions.

A memory grid is set up in a three-by-three format. This is the simplest version of it and provides for a recall of nine items. The initial activity used in Edu-Therapeutics is an unrelated picture/word association task. For this activity choose nine pictures of objects and nine noun cards. The object and the name card placed with it should not be related but should be able to be *associated*. The learner will be asked to make an association between the picture image and the word. The picture image will be placed on the learner's visual screen. Then the word will be turned into a visual image and the pictures will be combined in some functional or other related manner.

For instance, if the picture is *bread* and the word is *fingers*, the learner may choose to image the loaf of bread and then image fingers grasping the loaf.

If the picture is of a man's suit *coat* and the word is *money,* the learner may image the coat and then see money stuffed in the pocket and spilling out all over.

Benefits:

The learner is rehearsing several skills in this exercise: **concrete visualization, creative construction of visual imagery, attention, and practicing a memory strategy**. A sample activity grid is illustrated on the next page.

The Memory Grid exercise requires the learners to use their concrete imagery skills in retaining the picture. The use of the grid as a format is helpful because some of the memory appears to be related to *proximity*.

The grid provides a structure or organization for the information. The learner is then asked to perform a series of experiments with the grid. The experiments increase in difficulty and should be used over a series of sessions.

If too many experiments are used at one time, the learner will experience fatigue and stress. Both of these are to be conscientiously avoided.

Imaging Word - Picture Associations

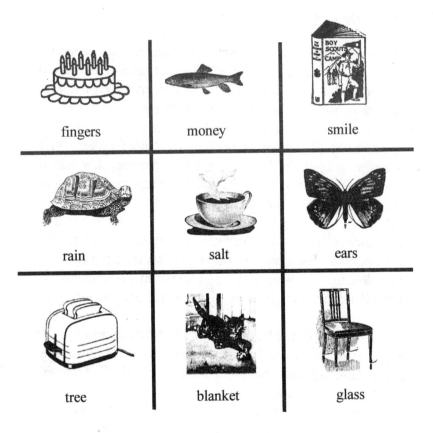

fingers	money	smile
rain	salt	ears
tree	blanket	glass

117

Responding to Confusion or Errors:

It is important for the therapist or teacher to be sensitive to the appropriate level for beginning the experiments. The learner should be at a level of challenge but not failure. It is the expertise of the therapist that provides this balance level.

When a learner cannot recall an association, a processing prompt may be provided first. [Cake/fingers: *Check your image of the picture on your screen, take a deep breath, let the word image join the picture.*] If the processing prompt does not work, then the therapist or teacher may be more specific with a questioning prompt. [Cake/fingers: *Check your image of the cake, take a deep breath, tell me what you see with the cake.*] If additional prompts are necessary, do a concrete prompt and display the two items. Ask then learner to re-image them. This is part of the concept of experimentation. Our expectations are not for perfect performance on every item every time. We are experimenting with learning a new strategy to understand what works best for each learner.

Experiment 1: *Recall words using picture stimulus.*

Once the learner has imaged each of the picture/word relationships, the words should be turned over but the pictures left exposed. Then ask the learner to go through the grid and recall the word and turn it over on the picture. If the learner can accomplish this task easily, ask them to collect the word cards, mix them up and then return them to the correct pictures, one at a time.

Experiment 2: *Recall pictures using word stimulus.*
The learner has imaged each of the picture/word relationships and now can turn over the pictures, leaving the words exposed. Ask the learner to identify the pictures that go with each of the words. If this is a comfortable task, then have the learner collect the pictures, mix them up and return them to the correct placement and the word card, one at a time.

Experiment 3: *Recall picture/word with proximity stimulus.*
Turn both the picture and word over. Ask the learner to identify both the picture and word using the grid to assist in recall. If this task is comfortable for the learner, increase the difficulty by having the learner collect the word cards and mix them, then collect the picture cards and mix them. Then ask him to replace the pictures and words to their original locations.

Experiment 4: *Tic -Tac-Toe game with memory grid.*
Explain to the learner that this 3X3 grid may be used as a Tic-Tac-Toe grid. Have the learner turn the pictures over to the blank side. Then play Tic-Tac-Toe with the learner by taking turns. In order to register an X or O in the box each player must identify the picture that belongs in the box.. When a player names the picture it should be turned face up, indicating the box has been chosen. [The learner and therapist

119

may find it most helpful, in the early stages, for the therapist to turn his/her choices one quarter turn to differentiate from the learner's choices.] The added pressure of trying to reason through the strategy to gain three in a row is an important memory stressor.

A Tic-Tac-Toe game can be played with numerous variations. If the identification of pictures is easy, then play with the words turned over and identify the words. For a more challenging task, turn both the picture and word over and require that they both be identified in order to choose a box.

The Tic-Tac-Toe game should be played with visual memory of where the X and O markers are located. If this is challenging to the learner, play the game without words or pictures on the grid. Just practice placing the markers through visual imagery on the chart. Once this is comfortable, the learner [and therapist or teacher] should image the grid on the wall or table and play the game without any actual written component. This provides excellent rehearsal for constructive visual memory.

Experiment 5: Extending Memory Skills
Rehearse recall of the picture and word associations with the learner. When the images appear to be comfortably retained, then collect the pictures and word cards and mix each set.

Place the set aside and wait for a thirty to fifty minute period before looking at them again. After the delay, have the learner look at the pictures and say the word that was associated with the picture. Then have the learner look at the word card and say the picture that was associated with the word.

Experiment 6: *Challenging Memory Skills*

Learners who have developed skills in association and memory may benefit from extending their competence. In order to challenge the learner on this series of tasks, a blank grid should be placed on the table. The boxes will need to be large enough for the learner to image a picture at least 2 X 2 inches.

Ask the learner to create an image of the object you say and place the image in the box. Make the objects common items with which the learner will be familiar. The therapist or teacher will need to record the items for reference. The recorded grid, which the learner will not view, might look like the one that follows:

CAT	TREE	SOFA
BOX	LAMP	BIRD
NAIL	HORSE	HAND

121

The learner will construct a visual image of the grid one picture at a time. When the objects have been imaged in each of the boxes, then review the grid by asking the learner to describe the image that was placed in each box. The activity of describing the picture to the therapist will reinforce the image for the learner and provide the teacher with a reference image.   [Use the Tic-Tac-Toe game for reinforcement and rehearsal.]

Once the pictures are imaged in place, a word card may be added to the grid. Ask the learner to integrate the picture with the image of the item on the word card.   Review the combinations by removing the word cards, mixing them and then giving them to the learner to place with the imaged pictures on the grid.

Pictures with Heard Word Cards
Place pictures on the grid and then say a word to go with each picture. Ask the learner to integrate the picture with the word to retain it. Be certain to record the words for teacher reference.

Ask the learner to collect the pictures and mix them up. Then place the pictures back in the original positions and say the word that has been assigned to each one. When this can be accomplished readily, ask the learner to collect the pictures or turn them over. Then have the learner say the picture and word for each position on the grid.

Using rehearsal and practice to extend our memory skills will increase our flexibility and effectiveness in using memory. It will improve the retention links in our memory pathways in our brains. Reinforce this image with the learner by talking about the areas in the brain that he or she is using for a task.

> *You are using several areas of your brain to accomplish this task. When you visualize the information you are activating the visual part of your brain [occipital area] and when you use your words to reinforce what you are seeing, you activate your verbal brain area [temporal]. The more areas you can activate the more likely you are to recall information. Enjoy the feeling of working with your whole brain. You are being very effective in extending its processing capability.*

Strategic Uses for Memory Grid
The Memory Grid may be used to learn numeric combinations such as times tables. In order to establish the grid the combinations should be discussed and worked out. The first Memory Grid which is memorized is the format grid. This provides a framework to use any set of combinations. It provides a reference point for the combinations. The

Numeric Grid should look like the following table:

1	4	7
2	5	8
3	6	9

In order to establish a Memory Grid for the 3X multiplication tables, the therapist or teacher will want to discuss what each combination means.   [*For instance: 3 X 3 means 3 sets of three. It is 3 + 3+ 3 = 9*] The discussion of the combination of numbers is helpful in creating an incentive for using the grid and the effort of memorizing the Memory Grid.   [*In order to avoid confusion in memory, no more than three grids should be used with the times tables unless the learner has exceptional memory skills.*]

The grid should be constructed with the combination:

3 X 1= 3	3 X 4 = 12	3 X 7 = 21
3 X 2 = 6	3 X 5 = 15	3 X 8 = 24
3 X 3 = 9	3 X 6 = 18	3 X 9 = 27

After the learner has recorded the information for each of the boxes in the grid the information should be simplified. Discuss with the learner the fact that they already know that 3 X would be in each box. Erase the 3X in each box. Then review with the learner that they know which number is represented in each box, from the numeric grid they had memorized first. Erase the numeral from the numeric grid in each box [and the equals sign!]

Now the box has just the sums [or answers] left to recall. The grid will look as follows:

3	12	21
6	15	24
9	18	27

In order to reinforce the memory of the grid, ask the learner to study the grid until she can image it on a blank wall. Have the learner fill in the blanks on a visualized grid. Point to the boxes randomly and have the learner report the number which would be in the box. Ask them to tell you what the number means...*i.e. What does the 12 stand for?... It means 3 X 4 equals 12.*

125

Play with the grid by writing the sums on cards and placing them on the form of the 3X3 grid. Then turn the card over and play Tic-Tac-Toe with the grid. The player has to recall the sum in order to choose the box as they play the game. This provides excellent reinforcement and rehearsal of the combinations.

This same strategy may be used for learning definitions, new words or studying for a matching type of test. Have the learner record the word on one card and the definition on another. Do the exercises from *Experiment 1, 2 and 3* to reinforce learning.

AUDITORY CONCEPTUALIZATION

The attribute of auditory conceptualization is important for comprehension both of heard and read information. In order to readily understand the information received in the verbal processing center of our brain we must associate it with prior information or a prior skill. For instance, if we are to understand the instructions by the postal clerk to "fill out the form for the passport application", we must relate the word "form" to the paper with the boxes and blanks that he has handed us. When the form asks for a "social security #" we need to have a reference that # equals number and we have to know our number or be able to look it up. In other words, we have a conception of these terms and can complete the task.

Learners who experience confusion with verbal input often have difficulty with both external and internal language retention. They may have inadequate vocabulary content. Often their auditory memory is inefficient or their processing has a time delay. By using activities to increase auditory concept development we extend our skills and learn to use this essential attribute effectively.

Benefits:

The learner is increasing several skills with these exercises and experiments: **extending auditory memory [listening retention], relating heard information to visual imagery, and attention.** These are all essential skills for enjoying reading, processing conversations readily, and maintaining a thought, while listening to someone else speak.

Auditory Conceptualization -Stimulus Cards

Stimulus cards are used by the therapist or teacher to increase the learner's auditory concept development. Prior to beginning the work with the cards, the images should be reviewed so that there is a consistent reference for the item. Review the concept of *inchness* or the length of an inch. Distinguish between rectangle and triangle and any other shapes which appear on the cards.

Experiment 7:   Provide the learner with a 3 X 5 card on which to record the image you will be dictating.   Give the instructions one shape at a time. Provide the location first, the shape second, and any unique attribute of the shape such as orientation, texture, or color last. Reference points such as top, bottom, corner, or clock placements are convenient for communicating locations.

Several sample card dictations are provided. Each shape or visual unit is described and then the learner is instructed to *draw it.* The therapist or teacher will want to develop a set of cards to use with instructions. These cards should include various levels of complexity.

Practice listening to the directions and filling-in the blank card.

Sample Card A:

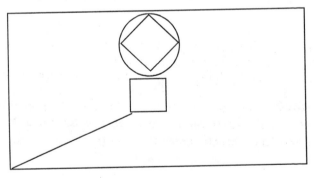

Description A: In the middle of the card, I see a square that is one half inch across. Draw it. Sitting on top of the square is a circle with a

128

diameter of one inch. Draw it. Inside the circle is a diamond shape. One point of the diamond is pointing straight up to the top, middle of the card. Draw it. There is a line goes from the bottom left corner of the square to the left corner of the card. Draw it.

Sample Card B:

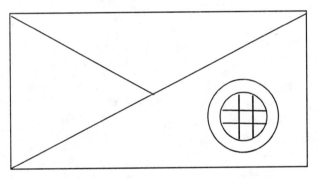

Description B: There is a line that extends from the top right corner of the card to the bottom left corner of the card. Draw it. There is a line that extends from the top left corner of the card to the middle point of the card. Draw it. One-half inch from the bottom right hand corner there is a circle with a diameter of one-half inch. Draw it. In the middle of the circle is a smaller circle with a diameter of one-fourth inch. The circle has a tic-tac-toe grid in the center of it. Draw it.

Sample Card C:

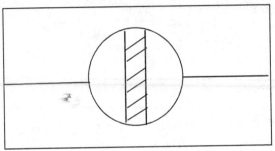

Directions C: In the center of the card there is a circle with a diameter of one inch. Draw it. From 9:00 on the clock rim to the left middle edge of the card there is a line. Draw it. From 3:00 on the clock rim to the right middle edge of the card there is a line. From 12:00 to 6:00 inside the circle there is a double line. Draw it. There are six stripes inside the double line that are oriented on a slant from 2:00 to 8:00. Complete the first stripe from the orientation and then add the other five at even intervals only inside the double line. Draw it. Fill in every other stripe to resemble a candy cane, beginning with the second stripe. Draw it.

These sample cards demonstrate varying degrees of difficulty. Preparing a collection of the cards saves time and energy, and assures that the therapist is consistent in giving the directions.

Increasing Level of Difficulty

When the learner can retain the location, shape and orientation for a single symbol unit, increase the difficulty by

130

giving instructions for two units. A learner who can retain two different items and their locations ,is ready to move into the next level of performance, which involves visualization of the card as it is being dictated.

Visualization Strategy for Recall
Finger Tracing Image
Ask the learner to look at the card as you describe a unit. Then have him trace where the image should appear with his finger, and anchor the image on the card. Continue with another unit. Ask the learner if the image is holding. If it is, then add another element. Continue the process until the learner signals that he needs to record the images. Have the learner draw over the units that have been traced on the card.

This activity will enable the learner to expand the capacity to recall information, and record and retain it while listening for additional information. This complex task is consistent with what we must do when we have to listen to directions or track a conversation while retaining information.

Visualization of Image
When the learner can retain with the tracing technique for anchoring, then the therapist can move to the next step. For this complex task, ask the learner to image each figure on the card without tracing it. Once the image is secured, add the next unit, and proceed in this manner until the learner signals

that she needs to record the image. Have the learner draw over the image that she sees on the card.

Imagery can be anchored effectively with these techniques. The more verbalization for reinforcement that the learner uses, the more likely the image will remain. The therapist will want to have the learner stop and describe what is on the card frequently, so that the verbalization process is effectively integrated.

We must be conscientious in telling the learners what they are doing and the strategy that they are using. It will then become part of their conscious language when they are making choices regarding how to do a task.

Auditory Conceptualization Using Stories:
Our focus in auditory conceptualization is on the skill of listening and retaining information.. The most effective retention of information takes place when it is recorded with multiple senses and locations in the brain. For instance, if we listen to directions and can image the streets and significant landmarks, we have used two different parts of our brain to record the instructions. If we also make hand gestures to reinforce the turn to the right or left as we see ourselves come to an intersection, we have added additional reinforcement through our kinesthetic recording in our brain.

The intent of the auditory conceptualization using stories, is to activate as many parts of the brain as possible in the effective registration of the information. This particular technique is subtle in its steps and the learner is often surprised by how effective it is with minimal effort. Since the steps in accomplishing the retention goal are very precisely designed, the learner moves simply by cooperating during the exercise.

During the first experience at each level, the learner may exhibit stress. Typically, the learner will need to be reminded to breathe and drink water to activate the circulation of the brain chemicals. When stress is noticed in a particular body region, such as a furrowed brow or a tense hand or foot, we reduce the demands of the task by unobtrusively altering the length of the phrases being used. A sample lesson from Mark's programming may provide a useful example:

> *JS - I am pleased with the selection you made. The cover of the book is so intriguing that it makes me want to read it. It provides a nice invitation.*

> *Mark - I have been wanting to read it and this will be a good opportunity.*

> *JS - I know you are curious about this exercise, so let me explain what we will be doing. Our goal is to*

increase your reading comprehension and allow you to enjoy your visualization of information as you read. It is also called "auditory conceptualization". In other words, it is the attribute that helps you hear something and recall it. That is the skill we will have when we are done with this series of exercises. Right now, I am going to ask you to do only what I tell you. If at some point you begin seeing images of what you are hearing, you can let me know. But, for now, I do not expect that you will be experiencing the images.

M - What am I supposed to do?

JS - I am going to read to you and ask you to repeat what I say.

M - That's all?

JS - Yes, just that simple. Let's start. "The boy's name was Santiago."

M - The boy's name was Santiago.

JS - "Dusk was falling as the boy arrived.."

M - Dusk was coming as he arrived..

JS - Take a breath and a sip of water. I see a furrow in your brow. Can you tell me what you are experiencing?

M - I am afraid I will forget what you are saying.

JS - I am certain that you will be comfortable in asking me if you miss something. It would make sense because it is your feedback that is directing me on this exercise.

At this point the length of the phrases being used was automatically altered to three or four units. It allowed Mark to begin to feel comfortable with the task.

Experiences in Listening

*Level One: T(Teacher) - **Read;** and L(Learner) -**Repeat***
Choose a story that is appropriate for the learner. The reading level for the story is unimportant but the interest level is critical. The story should have the potential for good imagery for the learner, and build on information from one session to the next.

Ask the learner to listen to the phrases as you read them and then to repeat after you. Assure them that you will work with the length of recall that is comfortable for them. You will know very quickly when the length is too long. The learner will appear stressed, will insert or alter words, or be unable to repeat the information. *Immediately adjust the length* of the phrase. It is the therapist or teacher's responsibility to assure that the learner is comfortable.

Sometimes the length of a phrase is longer than the learner can retain. It is appropriate to adjust the phrase although it may feel a bit awkward. For instance, if the listener was initially only comfortable with two words.... *"The boy's..."* / *"name was..."* / *"Santiago."* would be as appropriate for this purpose as longer phrases.

The listening /echo activity may continue for five to ten minutes. When the learner appears to fatigue it should be immediately terminated. It is not the amount of time that a learner spends on the activity, that is beneficial. It is the frequency of doing the activity, that is important. The learner should choose someone to assist with this experience so that he can practice four to five times each week.

The therapist will want to give a recap or review of the story prior to starting the exercise each day, such as a casual, *remember that Santiago is going to meet the merchant's daughter and is very excited about it.* Since we are not requesting comprehension of the learner, we make no assumption that he/she has recalled the information. Of course, during the next weeks of exercises at the different levels, the learner will *automatically* begin to comprehend the information. You can be observant for signs of this occurring, but must avoid any expectations. This is most effective when it is a *no expectation - i.e. no failure* task.

When to move to the next level:

The learner who is comfortable with the *listen/echo* level, should be recalling phrases of four to seven words with comfort. It is unlikely and unnecessary for the learner to retain complete sentences and there is no purpose in practicing to this level. Move to Level Two.

Level Two: **T- Read/Tap Syllables; and L - Echo/ Tap Syllables**

This task requires that, as therapist or teacher, you provide an example by reading the phrase and tapping the syllables in the words simultaneously. Then the learner will echo the phrase while tapping the syllables. Start the task with three-to-four word phrases again. Even if the learner is consistently doing longer phrases on Level One, return to the shorter phrase division until the learner is comfortable with the task.

This is a difficult task for most learners. The modeling that

137

you provide is critical for the learner, in understanding the syllable rhythm as it relates to the word. Most learners will make some errors, especially with multi-syllable words. These should be ignored unless the learner requests clarification. If there are numerous errors and the learner is unable to adapt to the task, it will be important to practice with the task of *syllable tapping*.

Practice Task for Syllable Tapping:

Use short phrases with one syllable words to begin the exercise.

> *I run.*
> *He thinks fast.*
> *She likes ice cream.*
> *The dog is big.*
> *The bird flies fast.*
> *The plane is full.*

Simple phrases with single syllable words should be used for the initial exercises. It may take several sessions to gain skill in the echo and tapping task with single syllable words. It is important to acquire this skill and is necessary to persevere. In the interim continue the story with Level One instructions.

When simple one-syllable phrases are comfortable, move to two-syllable words.

> *I like baseball.*
> *He plays football.*
> *She can cro/chet.*
> *The cat cha/ses me.*
> *The mouse scree/ches.*
> *The dog ran un/der the fence.*

Continue to increase the complexity of the words which are used in the phrases or sentences. When the learner is comfortable with the task of speaking and tapping, resume the Level Two activity. If necessary, at first, exaggerate the syllables in the words as you read them and use two-or-three word phrases to develop the learner's confidence.

It is essential that the learner practice this task frequently. Five to ten minutes, five times a week would be very beneficial in establishing this skill to an automatic level.

When the learner is unable to have assistance in practice, a tape can be prepared which has time delays, for the learner to repeat and tap the phrases after listening to them. The auditory reception of the tapping on the tape, is slightly more difficult because the visual resources are unavailable for imitation.

We frequently ask the learner to tap while they are talking on the phone or privately tap the words they are thinking. This will establish the pattern of associating words and their syllable count. Of course they will sound somewhat stilted initially as they talk because they are thinking about the syllable count as they are talking. Over a period of time they will develop good fluency with it.

Level Three: **T - Read/ Tap; and L - Repeat (inner-voice)/Tap**

There are several different ways of moving the learner to the next level. Any of these will work and they should be chosen based on the progression skill of the learner. For a fragile learner, the sequence should include all of the steps described in order to achieve this level. An example of the steps is described in the dialogue:

> *JS - We are going to change the task this time because you are becoming too adept at doing it. After all it won't be much fun if its too easy!*
>
> *Lucy -I know you want to make me miserable and keep me suffering!*
>
> *JS - That's progress! This time I will continue to read to you and you will echo what I am saying. We*

will tap out the syllables. The difference is, I would like for you to whisper your echo as you are tapping the syllables. Okay?

L - That's it? I can do that.

JS - Let's start..

The purpose of this task will be to gradually fade the external voice of the learner. We will go through several levels of prompting the fade. The first level will be for the learner to whisper and tap what they are hearing. The second level will be to have the learner *mouth* the words or *repeat it without the voice*. The therapist will be able to see, by observing the learner's lips that the words are being recorded. The therapist will also hear the syllables and be able to track the sequence of taps for the content.

After practicing with Lucy for several weeks with the whispered echo response, she was ready to move to the next level.

JS - We are going to change the task by removing the whisper. I will say and tap it, you will mouth and tap it. Sometimes we call this "voiceless talking". In other words, I can see your mouth moving and if I can lipread I will know what you are saying. Do you have

141

any questions?

L - Is this hard?

JS - It might be hard for some students but I think you are ready for it because you have mastered all the other steps and are powerful in taking new ones. It may feel strange at first but you can do it.

L - Let's start.

This level is an important transition point because the learner is now having to use an *inner voice* for certain. The voice is no longer external and in order for the brain to *hear* it , it will use internal language.

Obviously, the next step will be to have the learner only use internal language. They will stop mouthing the words and will just tap the syllables. This was very comfortable for Lucy at this point, but many learners need to move slowly with this level, because they are *just developing* an awareness of their inner voice and its use.

JS - Okay, we are ready for our next level. You have moved quickly during the last two weeks with this. Have you been working on it at home?

142

L - My mother makes me do it every morning. It's actually okay, though. We are reading a good story and I like it.

JS - Your mom must love you a lot. Not only is she showing you that you are a fast learner but she's making it pleasant. She is going to like doing the next level.

L - What are we going to do differently?

JS - This time you will listen to her read and tap the story and you will just have to tap it back. What do you think will be happening with your voice?

L - I don't have to use it?

JS - No such luck! You get to use it inside your head, just like you were thinking it or hearing it in your brain. Actually, it is this part of the brain (temporal lobe) that will be echoing it for you. If I had a listening-scope that could listen to the voice inside your brain, I would hear you repeating it! That would be very handy for me wouldn't it?

At this point the learner is practicing using the inner voice for recording information. We are moving into the retention of auditory information and will begin experiencing conceptualization during the next few levels.

Level Four: *T- Read; and L - Tap*

The intent at this stage is to phase out the syllable tapping model that the therapist has provided. It is likely that the learner is completely comfortable with syllable tapping. If for any reason the exercises at Level Two were not sufficient, they should be repeated and rehearsed until competency is apparent. The therapist will use continued syllable tapping at this point, to know that the learner is actually echoing the information sufficiently.

The learner is most likely finding that he/she is tracking the story by now. They will appear to be recognizing the characters and laughing or reacting to what is happening in the story. The therapist will resist the urge to start quizzing the learner about the story!

Level Five: *T- Read; and L - Echo (inner voice)/ tap periods*

The syllable tap is phased out at this level. Instead the learner is instructed to echo the sentence and then tap twice. This is consistent with the punctuation tapping used for Neurological Impress Reading referenced in *"You Don't Have to Be*

144

Dyslexic". The therapist will want to read in complete sentences to see if the learner can retain the information.

As the learner is tapping at the end of the sentence, he may begin to experience considerable comprehension. When the therapist is reviewing the story at the beginning of the session, the learner may insert information or choose to do the recapping of the story himself.

Level Six: T - Read; and L - Image/Tap

The final phase of auditory conceptualization training actually has the learner comprehending what he or she is hearing. The therapist instructs the learner to listen, and then image or relate the information he has heard.   When he has the information, he should tap twice and the therapist will continue with the next sentence.

Some of the sentences will not create new images, and it is important to relieve the learner from the expectation that he or she will be receiving constant images and that the images will be *like a movie*.   Imagery is not actually like a movie, although the experience is satisfying in the same way as experiencing a movie.   It is important to relieve the learner's expectations.

It is appropriate to begin by asking the learner to share his or her image. This will provide you with information regarding what he or she is experiencing. Mark was especially excited about his images as he experienced them.

> *Mark - I don't mean to laugh at this activity but I am so delighted with what I am experiencing, I am happy and want to laugh.*

> *JS - You are experiencing...*

> *M - It is really no effort at all. I can hold the information and it is not a panic feeling. I don't say to myself "I'm not getting this." anymore. Its like it really isn't any problem to know what its about.*

> *JS - You will begin noticing it in other areas, too. Like when you are in a conversation with someone, you will just know what they are saying. I suspect that you have been experiencing that already.*

> *M - It's true, last week I was in this meeting and it was like, I just knew what was going on and it was easy to respond. None of my emotions were getting in the way even though it was a really emotional meeting.*

> *JS - I would like to see you rehearsing at home*

between our sessions. Could you choose some light novel that you could read? It should be something simple with good imagery. Agatha Christy writes some wonderful scenes. You feel like you are there in England. Her characters are not quite so clear but the surroundings really are vivid. If you don't want to read for yourself, then borrow story tapes from the library and listen to them. You can sit back and shut your eyes and enjoy the imagery.

Free Tasks

During the sessions on auditory conceptualization it is useful to do *free tasks*. These are times when you read a short story to the learner just for fun. At first they will be suspicious that you are going to quiz them about it or make them do an exercise.

> *JS - I would like to share a quick story with you, just for fun. Sit back and relax and just enjoy it.*
>
> *M - What do you want me to do?*
>
> *JS - Nothing special, just enjoy yourself.*

The entire time we read the story the first time, the learner is watching carefully and trying to remember the information.

> *JS -....."and the farmer picked up his new truck and drove away with a smirk on his face and pride in his heart."*

> *M - What do you want me to do now?*

> *JS - Nothing, I just thought you would enjoy it.*

> *M -You mean I didn't have to do anything but enjoy it.*

> *JS - Right. Perhaps we will have time to do another one next time.*

> *M - I'd like that. I could just listen and relax.*

Our learners are so accustomed to working hard at everything and being responsible for responding, that they need experiences that are without energy cost! Skill in auditory conceptualization gives the learner the feeling of control over the verbal environment. It creates comfort and a feeling of power. It is a new experience for learners who have not felt empowered in this area before. Success in this area is absolutely key in establishing a base for performing effectively in school, work and interpersonal relationships.

VISUAL CONCEPTUALIZATION

The attribute of visual conceptualization is best described as the skill in seeing something and being able to verbalize it. It is the ability to communicate what one sees or experiences. Inefficiency in this attribute is usually observed as a difficulty in verbal expression. A learner will be unable to share or communicate what she has experienced, or may find it difficult to give verbal directions to a place that she can drive to easily.

It is this attribute which contributes to skill in writing. Learners who use it easily can verbally describe information and write it, because they can image what is happening, or can visually image an outline or sequence of presentation. Good speakers often possess this skill. It allows them to visually plan as they are presenting, to visually analyze the audience response, and transfer that into their language system.

Speakers with inefficiency in this area will observe an audience member looking confused or disinterested and send it to their feeling response level. The feeling level then sends the language of *"Oh, they don't like me. What will I do now?"* in other words, a panic response.

149

Individuals with good visual conceptualization will instead, observe the audience response and adjust the content, or respond on an intellectual rather than emotional level. The inner language will probably sound more like... *"Oh, they look disinterested. I will switch to an area that will interest them, and then return to this area at a later point in my presentation."* They can visually image the content and manipulate it as they are speaking with minimum interruption.

In order to establish skill in visual concept development, it will be essential to meld the skills of visualization and verbal inner-language. If either of these is a primary issue it will be important to begin resolution prior to attempting to use the areas for integrated functioning. For instance, if visual memory is difficult for the learner, it should be established at a five-digit level minimum before attempting these exercises.

Periodically in presenting information about visualization, we find individuals who claim to be unable to visualize. If they are able to read or spell, they are recording visual imagery although they may not recognize it as such. They could not recognize the image of a word if they had no visual imagery. Most likely they are victims of the perfectionist symptoms and think that they need to see an image vividly and in a solid form. It is rare that we can experience these types of images. Most of the time we need to concentrate on them, and embellish them with language to construct a detailed image, as we discussed in *Getting the Image, Visual Imagery as an Attribute.*.

The exercises to establish visual conceptualization skills tend to be very simple in nature. The simpler the task the more likely it is exercising and stimulating those brain areas in which we want to establish efficiency in learning. The initial task uses the stimulus cards from the *Auditory Conceptualization* training.

Visual Conceptualization - Stimulus Items

A stimulus may be any picture, object or Stimulus Card with shapes or items. The learner will be asked to describe the item to the therapist. Initially, the therapist will model the task to the learner.

> *JS - We are going to do a different task today. We want to expand your visual conceptualization skills. In order to do this, we have to exercise the visual and language parts of your brain. The visual cells in your brain will register what I show you, and then you will put it into words by activating your language cells.*
>
> *I will show you how to do this first and then ask you to do it. I am going to choose an object in the room and describe it to you. Cover your eyes or turn away*

151

and I will select something I can see behind you.

L - Do you care if I have my eyes open?

JS - That is a good question. You can choose how you want to do it. I know that you can image with your eyes open. I just don't want you staring at what I am describing.

Let's do one. I see an object that is about six inches high. It is a female figure. It is made of terra-cotta clay and is that adobe-like color. The figure is seated on the ground. She has black hair and a turquoise top and black skirt. Are you imaging it? Can you tell me what you are seeing?

L - Yep, it's an Indian lady sitting on the ground. She is made out of clay stuff and her hair and skirt are both black.

JS - Good job. I have a few more details I want you to have. She is holding an armful of five children and a book. She is reading the book to the children.

L - I know, it's the story teller doll.

JS - Good, but let's orient where she is on the shelf so

152

you will recognize her when you look for her.   She is on the first shelf of the book case nearest the door. She is on the left side of the shelf and there are books on the rest of the shelf. Do you have it?

L - Yes, I know right where she will be.

JS - Do you know how she is oriented on the shelf yet?

L - Yes, well no, I'm not sure. Did you tell me?

JS - No, I haven't. Are there any other questions you will have? [L shakes head, no]. Okay, her feet point to the books on the shelf and we mostly see her from her right side.

Now that the task has been modeled, the therapist will ask the learner to do the same thing. We will have the learner do a series of exercises to establish this skill. The task will require a great many prompts in the beginning.

Exercise One: **Visual description of Object**

First, have the learner choose an object without telling you what it is. Then have her tell you how to orient yourself so that you cannot see the area where the object is in the room or cover your eyes.

Ask the learner to describe the object in her own words so that you can see the object. Tell her that she will be creating the *image in your brain* with *her words.*

You might say... *Choose an object in the room and describe it to me so that I will recognize what it is. I may need to ask questions so that I can image it more effectively. I will cover my eyes so I can't actually see it.*

Allow the learner to tell you as much as she can about what she is seeing. Whenever she pauses, use your words to give her feedback on what you are picturing. You will be modeling how to picture information. It is helpful to verbalize as much as you can about what you are doing.

> *JS - I am imaging a picture on the first shelf of the cabinet. I think that you have placed the picture on the left side of the shelf. It seems to be a picture of four people but I don't have a clear image of the people yet, can you help me with that?*
>
> *L - There are two ladies and two men. They are standing up and smiling at us.*
>
> *JS - I see two ladies and two men but I don't know where to put them yet... tell me more.*

*L - Oh, one of the ladies is on the left side and then
there is a man and the other lady and then the other
man on the right. Okay?*

*JS - Good, I have them in order...(gesturing) a lady,
man, lady, and a man. Tell me more so I can see them
clearly.*

This type of dialogue sequence provides modeling for the
learner in understanding how her words are communicating
with the listener. It is likely that this first exercise will need
to be repeated for several sessions, before the learner begins
to take the visual image and put it into words with more
confidence. In the next exercise we will provide structure to
the process.

Exercise Two: *Visual Description Using Attribute Guide*

Once we have an opportunity to hear the verbalization skills
accompanying the first exercises, then we want to begin to
give structure to the task. An Attribute Guide is introduced
to provide the stimulus needed for good description. Each
attribute card is introduced to act as a guide to determine
when the description is completed. We often like to model
the use of the attribute cards for the learner. This process
provides a model of using a strategy for performing a task.

ATTRIBUTE   GUIDE

LABEL	MAJOR PARTS
COLOR	QUANTITY
COMPOSITION	COMPARISON
SIZE	CATEGORY
SHAPE	PHYSICAL ATTRIBUTES
FUNCTION or ACTION	LOCATION

L - Label, you told me what it was. I think you said a female figure. Major parts, I'm not sure if you used that one. Color, that was for sure, you said it was clay colored and the color of her clothes and hair. I knew it was made out of clay so you must have told me the composition. Is that right?

JS - Good, composition means what something is made of. It's different from the other kind of composition which means.

L - To write something!

JS - Yes, you knew that. What other attributes did I use?

L - I know you told me about the location. I don't think we talked about category or shape or size.

JS - What could I have said that would have given you information about category?

L - Would it be like a decoration or art thing?

JS - What other objects would be in the category of decoration?

157

L - Oh, a picture or a vase or flowers on the shelf.

JS - Then I think it would definitely be in that category. You tested the attribute of category and decided it met the test. You checked it against other items of the same type. That's a good strategy.

Once you have modeled how you used the attribute guide cards, then choose four to six of them and put them on the table in front of the learner. You can adjust the degree of difficulty on this task, by varying the information which you provide to the learner and the complexity of the stimulus. For younger or more involved learners, use a single object placed in front of the learner. For older or skilled learners use a picture with a variety of components. This is also the progression used in increasing difficulty as a learner progresses on the exercise. Generally the degree of difficulty is associated with the complexity of the stimulus material. For instance, the beginning level might be a simple, common object like a pencil or a cup. Then complexity might be increased by adding two items together like a spoon in the cup. A more complex object can be used next like a telephone or toy with several parts. The next level of difficulty is to move to pictures or drawings of objects. The same progression can be used with pictured items and finally, complex pictures like scenery or events.

158

We have demonstrated how we used the attribute guide in our own descriptions, and now we are going to ask the learner to use several of the attribute cards in a description. Place an object in front of the learner and ask him to describe it using the guide cards. When he has used one of the cards, like the label card, reach over and turn it face down. When each of the cards has been turned over, pause and reinforce the learner's use of the cards... *Good use of the attributes.*

Next ask the learner to turn them over again one at a time, and tell you what the attribute was that he had mentioned. If he cannot recall it, provide a prompt...*I thought you said that the lady was made of clay...that is a good composition word. It tells us what something is made of. Would you agree or should we add something else?*

This exercise should be completed a number of times, until the learner is adept at describing complex pictures and using attributes as a guide in the descriptions. It will become an effective strategy for the learner to implement, for both written and verbally-presented work.

Visual conceptualization will be used in the exercises for developing written expression. It is important to develop skill in visual conceptualization prior to implementing the writing skill training.

159

WRITING AS A VISUAL-VERBAL PROCESS

I can't think of anything to write. Where do I start. I don't know what to say... sound familiar? This has always been the chant of students when they receive a writing assignment. Unfortunately, it is what learners believe. When they are focusing their language on *I can't* statements, their language center is engaged and can not possibly be used to find a solution. They are stuck in their emotional verbalizations.

In order to disengage the emotional connection in writing, it is necessary to change the task considerably. For this purpose we teach a series of steps (strategies) to produce written work. At the early levels, the learner uses a process which readily facilitates positive, productive language.

The process of writing requires the use of both verbal and visual conceptualization skills. For some learners an image appears first, and then they describe it or elaborate on it with words - visual conceptualization. Other learners discuss it with their inner language and then construct word images or outlines. Both of these strategies are effective. The techniques described in the visual-verbal writing process will allow the learners to develop their own strengths.

Developing Attribute Guides - Step One

These activities will use the attribute guide and cards. We like to begin with an attribute activity in which we write as many descriptive or category words as we can think of on cards. Words might include: red, blue, green, large, small, soft, hard, smooth, sleek, plastic, wood, cotton, metal, organic, flesh, round, square, triangular, bigger, smaller, prettier, side, right, left, top, work, write, draw, erase, and many others. Then we make category cards including: color, size, composition, shape, comparison, parts, and purpose.

We place the category cards across the top of the table and then ask the learner to place the descriptive words under the most appropriate category. When we have finished, the table is filled with words under each category.

> **Color:** red, blue green, yellow, brown, black, white.
> **Size:** large, small, thin, long, tall, short, fat, huge.
> **Composition:** Description of... soft, hard, slick, rough, sticky, smooth, sleek, jagged. Content of... plastic, wood, lead, flesh, fur, organic, man-made, metal, water.
> **Shape:** Round, square, triangular, rectangular, straight, moon shaped.
> **Comparison:** Bigger than, prettier, smaller, fatter, taller, rougher, smoother, slicker.

161

Parts: handle, stock, trigger, top, bottom, side, knob, keys, pegs.

Function or Purpose: Work, play, dig, write, repair, erase, transport, beautify.

To demonstrate how to use the descriptive words, we choose an object and ask the learner to select the words in each of the categories which could be used to describe the object. For instance, if the object is a pencil, under color they might select yellow, silver, black and brown. Each of the characteristics is included on a chart to assist in vocabulary development. An example follows:

COLOR	SIZE	COMPOSITION	SHAPE	COMPARISON	PARTS	PURPOSE
yellow	long	wood	round	fatter than pen	point	write
silver	skinny	lead			sides	work
black - lead		metal			eraser	draw
brown - eraser		rubber				erase

This exercise should be repeated using a variety of different objects or pictures. Once the learner has selected the descriptors from the cards, ask if he would like to add any other descriptors that are not on the cards, but might be appropriate for the item.

The learner should do this activity easily with the cards, before attempting to move into a structured writing activity. Some learners spend several weeks at this level while others spend only a session.

Writing a Description - Step Two

Now that learners can use a variety of words to describe an object, they are ready to begin writing a description. Give them the Attribute Guide and word cards, and ask them to choose the words they would use to describe *a pencil* or whatever is appropriate for the learner. If you are working with a novice writer, these steps are quite appropriate.

Once learners have a vocabulary to work with, in creating a description, they can put the words into sentences. Have them begin by making a sentence for each of the attributes. First have them use the noun...*The pencil is*...and then use the pronoun... *It is*...

> *The pencil is blue.*
> *It is yellow.*
> *It is silver.*
> *It is wood...etc.*

Once this task is easy and comfortable, then teach learners how to combine sentences.

It is yellow.   + It is silver.   = It is yellow and silver.

Sentence combining is a difficult task for new writers and young children. You may need to review it for several sessions. Consider doing the exercises verbally and keep the written work to a minimum if it is difficult.

Next, teach learners to use the adjectives in front of the noun, and practice with the sentences they have been using in the original exercise...

The pencil is yellow.   It is blue.   It is made of wood.
The yellow and blue pencil is made of wood.

Give the learner numerous verbal exercises to rehearse this type of sentence combining. When the task is completed easily, then they can begin to write the sentence that has been created. It is important for the learners to make the connection between verbal language and written language.

Once learners can easily do sentence combining they are ready to do a descriptive paragraph of an object. If they appear to have difficulty or be hesitant, start them with an object they have already described during their verbal and written exercises.

As a therapist or teacher, you will be most effective if you can move learners in small successful steps, and gradually reinforce them with statements reflecting on their good independent skills.

> *JS - It feels to me like you are comfortable with the descriptive guide words and combining them for fancy sentences.*

> *L - Yep, this is easy, not like really having to write something.*

> *JS - Of course, you are "writing something"!*

> *L - You know what I mean, it feels okay.*

> *JS - Then you are really going to feel good about doing the next step. It always helps when you have mastered it before you start. I really like the way you made interesting sentences out of the attribute words. Have you noticed that you are using them when you are talking about things or describing something?*

> *L - I don't know.*

> *JS - Let's check it out. Here is a pencil. Go through your cards and choose the attribute words you would use and put them in front of you. Then give me a description of the pencil.*

> *L - Okay, Here goes... I have a red and black pencil. It has stripes and it is new. It is bigger than my old pencil. It has lead and writes dark.*

> *JS - Look at the pencil and remember your description. Now let's write it down. I will be your dictionary. Tell me any word that you need spell-check for. Otherwise, I will be very quiet and not interrupt you as you talk it through with your inner voice.*

> *L - I did it! This is easy. Can I do another one?*

It is efficient to dialogue with our inner voice in writing. We can almost hear it dictate to us what we would like to say. It is this skill in dialoguing that brings confidence to writing.

Incentive Activity: For younger students or classes, allow them to collect points for each attribute they use. We usually give one point for attributes in the color, shape and size column, and two points for each attribute from the composition, comparison, parts or purpose categories. This encourages learners to utilize the descriptive words. The points can be charted... That's a twenty-point paragraph! Asking the learners to focus on the attribute words as they are counting them, removes the focus from the stress of writing and places it on the description components.

Describing a picture or event - Step Three

Now that preparing a description is comfortable, we apply the skill to describing a picture or event. Prepare an Attribute Guide with the appropriate categories across the top, and then place attribute cards under each category. For instance, if the picture was of a mountain scene, you might select the categories of color, scent, size, for instance:

COLOR	SCENT	SIZE
green	pine	massive
yellow	fresh	spindly
brown		huge

You will want to select all the categories and spend time developing the vocabulary that relates to the picture or event. This may be the activity for a single lesson if it is difficult for the learner.

When writing, it is appropriate to spend time thinking about the subject. It is an important strategy to teach learners. It is not essential to do all the parts to a task at once. It is often beneficial to prepare to do the task and then spend time cogitating!

JS - You have developed a wonderful vocabulary. I almost feel like I am in the picture when I think about these words. Are there any others you want to add?

L - There are plenty here to use. That was a lot of work to make that many words.

JS - I am impressed by how many words you had in your head! I am surprised they aren't oozing out your ears!

L - Right! (Big smiles). Now am I going to have to start writing them?

JS - No, actually I want you to cogitate for a bit about them.

L - What? I don't think I know how to do that.

JS- Cogitate? (Nods.) It means to think about something, to ponder it, or to really spend some time letting it sink in. That is what I want you to do with this writing. Take the picture with you and I will preserve your words, and we will do the writing next time. It is always important to give yourself time to let it settle in. You will think about it when you look at the picture, but don't work on it. Just play with it occasionally.

When preparing to write from a picture or event, it is important to organize the attribute cards. Once all the words that apply to the picture have been identified, they will need to be sorted to relate to general or specific items in the picture or event. For instance, if the following words had been selected to relate to a picture of a mountain scene with a lake, the chart may look like this:

COLOR	SIZE	TEXTURE	SHAPE	MOOD	COMPARISON
dark green	massive	slick	round	warm	bigger than
red	skinny	rough	straight	peaceful	taller ..
blue	tall	smooth	rectangle	still	smoother..
dark brown	huge	jagged	oval	relaxed	powerful..

Learners and therapist together can brainstorm words that describe the picture. It is a wonderful time for introducing new vocabulary words. Bring out the Thesaurus and look up words to add to the selection.....*If we like "massive" what other words would mean the same...let's look it up..."huge, heavy, cumbersome"... Should we add any of these to our list?*

Once we have a good selection of vocabulary words, then we have the learners begin to group them into descriptions of specific parts of the picture. For instance, the learners will select the words that would describe the pine trees (tall, furry, green, brown) or the mountain (rough, round, bigger than..majestic, still peaceful).

Ask the learners to verbalize sentences which describe the picture using the word cards, and place the word cards in the sequence they are used. These will serve as a prompt for writing. At first, learners are likely to return to the noun/verb format, but let them verbalize them as they wish. As therapist or teacher, you may want to record what they are saying.

By having the learners verbalize the sentences you have heard what their writing will look like. It is much easier to correct it before it is written than after, so provide the prompts in the sentences now. For instance, if you recorded: *The mountain is dark. The mountain is round. The mountain is majestic,* you may want to give a prompt about sentence combining or using a pronoun. Rather than making a criticism, ask

170

questions... *Have you thought about using your sentence-combining skills on any of the sentences?... When you made the sentences before, you used the noun and sometimes replaced it with a pronoun. Will you choose to use that, in this writing?*

This is a good time to introduce using a descriptor as an adjective, by placing it in front of the noun. Learners do not have to have an elaborate discussion of the parts of speech. They will learn them more easily if they are just used as references while you are working....*Let's use the adjective, the descriptor word, "dark", in front of the noun, the namer in that sentence.* Show the learners how to combine sentences using the adjective/noun combination such as:

> *The mountain is dark. + The mountain is majestic.*
> *= The dark mountain is majestic.*
> *The pine tree is tall. + The pine tree is furry.*
> *= The tall pine tree is furry.*

As the learners are preparing to write the descriptive paragraph, we like to ask them to place themselves in the picture for a few minutes. You can ask them to *surround themselves with the picture*, experience it all around them. Ask them to establish a perspective for their visualization. Where are they in the picture; what do they see, feel, smell. Are they gaining anything that they did not think of, when

171

they were outside just looking at the picture? Ask them to tell you what they are seeing. Use a scribe, or tape the descriptions, to keep for the written task. You will be aware of the learner using the vocabulary from the attribute exercises such as in this selection:

> *I am sitting under a furry pine tree. The pine tree is taller than an office building. I can look up at a mountain. It is rough and round. It is still and peaceful on the mountain. The dark mountain is majestic.*

Once learners can verbalize a paragraph, they can begin recording it in writing. It will be helpful to remind them that they are using their inner voice to verbalize the information to write, and that it is a very effective way of writing.

Using a Format for a Simple Composition - Step Four

Learners who experience difficulty in knowing what to write, and how to begin, benefit from format writing. Prior to using this technique, learners should be skilled in writing descriptions as in the previous exercises.

We use a W-Guide Form to assist in developing the content for this strategy. The form is just a simple grid as follows:

WHO	WHEN	WHERE	WHAT

Guide the learners by providing or helping them choose content for the composition. By combining the Story Imaging Technique and this activity, you will have appropriate content for writing.

Story Imaging Technique - Step Five

The Story Imaging Technique develops a learner's skill in using visualization for recalling information. The training technique is a rather simple process in visualization or imagery. It relies on and expands visual memory skills, integrates verbal and visual information, and assists in content storage for long-term retrieval.

The therapist or teacher gives the learner a sentence which contains specific information. Then the therapist guides the learner in creating and anchoring a visual image of the information. This was a very powerful technique for our learners who participated in this series.

> *JS - Let's do a visualization activity from listening input. We are going to do the story of Rosa Parks. I would like you to anchor each of the sentences as you*

173

hear them. We will create the first box on the face of the door over there. I would like you to anchor in some manner that there was an African-American child born in 1914 and her name was Rosa. How could you image this?

M - I see a hospital room, you mean like that?

JS - Sure, this is your image.

M - I see a nursery where there are a bunch of babies and I see a man and woman who are looking through the window.

JS - How have you anchored the date?

M - On the front of the baby's crib, there is a chart and the date 1914 is written on the chart.

JS- May I continue? (Nod) Place the next picture on the top shelf of the far book case. The statement is..Black children and white children could not go to school together.

M - Do I have to connect it to the image over there? (No), Okay, then I see two different school houses, side by side, like Little Red School houses and I see a

174

line of white children going into one and a line of black children going into the other.

JS - They could not use the same drinking fountain. Let's put this one on the second shelf.

M - I see a drinking fountain in front of the school where the white children are going in, and hanging on the drinking fountain is a black child's face with a ghost buster sign across it.

JS - On the third shelf...They could not sit in the same part of the bus.

M - I see the bus pulls up at school and the white children get in and sit in the front of the bus and then the black children get in and sit at the back.

JS - Okay, now Rosa...

M - There is more?

JS - Oh, yes, we have this whole room to fill. Are the images staying? Check them in their frames . Can you recall them?

M - Yes, they are there.

175

JS - Rosa was a very good student in school.

M - Is this the same Rosa? (Yes) How do I know that? Maybe I should put her name in one of the frames.

JS - Good idea, where would you put it?

M - In the first frame, right on the chart with her birthdate.   So, I see a little girl going into the school, and it is after all the other children are gone, but she is still working hard.

JS - When she was nineteen she married Raymond Parks.

M - I see a beautiful wedding, she was nineteen.. How do I anchor that... I know I could put it on her wedding dress, embroider it on!

JS - Even though she had graduated from high school, Rosa could only get a job sewing for people.

M - I see her sitting and sewing.

JS - Give me a review of your images and point to the picture location on the wall as you describe them to me.

M - I see an incubator with the name Rosa and the date 1914 on the foot of it. I see two schools and an image of a water fountain with a sign on it forbidding drinking except by the white children. I see a little girl in the school house who is studying very hard. I see the marriage picture and then her sitting sewing in her house.

JS - Now can you give me five pieces of information about Rosa Parks using language.

M - Rosa Parks was born in 1914. She went to school and studied hard. She had to go to a separate school from the white children and could not drink at the same drinking fountain. She got married to a man named Parks. Even though she had a high school degree, the only job she could get was sewing for people in her home.

JS - Good recall. You have both the facts and the sequence correct. How does it feel?

M - I love it. I really want to catch up on my history and this would be a useful way of learning it.

The technique of imaging factual information and then reviewing the images is very powerful for recall. There are several other steps that are effective with this which make it quite utilitarian.

> *JS - Just for a moment I would like to have you look at the pictures again, but this time I want you to see them in your mind. If you are comfortable with it, please close your eyes. See the door and the image you have on it?*

> *M - Yes, it is there, I can see the shelves and all the pictures.*

> *JS - Good. Now look at the first picture and then add your imagination, see her growing up and going to school. See the different schools and the children moving about... fast forward...see her go to the water fountain and then walk away and go back to the one near her school... fast forward...see her studying hard in her school house and graduating from high school...fast forward... what is next?*

> *M - She is marrying Raymond Parks and then she is sewing and can't get a job except that.*

It is obvious that this process is readily anchored in the mind's eye and memory. The learner feels quite in control and comfortable with the process. If you wanted to prove it to the learner, you could have them look at the pictures in the reverse order and tell her life from end to beginning.

The next step is adding language to the process. In order to do this, we ask the learners to make as many boxes on a piece of paper as there are pictures on the wall. Then we ask them to take the first image off the door and place it in the first box. Once they can see the image in the box, we ask them to choose a word (or two) that best describes the picture and write it on the box..

> *JS - The next step will be for you to place the image from the wall onto this paper. Let's create enough boxes on the paper for each of your images. Then take the image and place it in the first box.*

> *M - I did it. I have the image of the nursery scene in the box.*

> *JS - Now, choose a word that best describes the scene and write it on the box.. You can use more than one if you wish.*

> *M - Okay, incubator and 1914. (Writes words in box.)*

> *JS - Continue to do this with each of the images, transfer them to the paper in the box and then label*

179

the box. (Writes them in each box.) I see...schools, water fountain, studying, bus, married - Parks- 19, and sewing.

See how you have anchored this information. You can anchor any type of information this way. You could then use these prompts to help you study or remember the information. It works for an essay, true- false test, or multiple choice. You can choose the subject, anchor the images, label the images and then just recall from it. For instance, give me the words without looking at the piece of paper except in your memory.

M - Incubator - 1914, schools, water fountain, studying, bus, married-Parks-19, and sewing. I can't believe how easy that was.

JS - Of course, you don't want to go around for the rest of your life recalling this particular piece of information, but if you were giving a lecture about civil rights, it would be important to recall. The important piece here is that you just demonstrated your power to hear, read, and learn something.

M - Yeah, feels good.

The Story Imaging Technique and recording of prompt words provides an excellent vehicle for improving writing with the W-Guide. Use the following steps to develop the story content:

1. Develop the content for a composition by presenting the information and having the learner build an image of the information. Anchor each image in a separate place on the wall in a sequential manner.

2. Construct and discuss the image for each important event. (Story Imaging Technique).

3. Have the learner describe the images and choose a word or phrase for each of the images. (Anchor with words.)

4. Ask the learner to hold the image of the word/s on the picture, and verify the recall by having the learner point to the image location and provide the key word.

5. Discuss the W-Guide with the learner and ask them to fill in the grid with the information.

For example, if we were going to develop a W-Guide for the information for Alexander Graham Bell it might look like the grid on the following page. It has been filled in with the important details to be included in the descriptive paragraph.

181

Alexander Graham Bell - An Important Man

WHO	WHEN	WHERE	WHAT
Alexander Graham Bell	1845	Scotland	Born
Grandfather	1860	England	Visited Inventor's Museum
Parents: Father			Teacher for deaf students
Mother			Deaf
Alexander	1870	United States	Teacher/ Inventor
Tom Watson			Friend, Helped invent telephone
	1876		Received patent for phone.

6.   Provide the subjects with several colors of highlighter pens. Ask the learner to highlight in yellow the two or three most important words on the chart. (*Alexander Graham Bell, telephone.*)   This will constitute the information for the *topic sentence.* Assist the learners in verbalizing a   sentence or several different ones and then record the one they wish to use.... *Alexander Graham Bell was an important man because he developed the telephone.*

You can assist the learners in adding relevancy to the subjects with prompting questions like: *What do you mean by important? ...What was the impact of telephones?... What would have been different today without the telephone?* ...just general questions to develop vocabulary and concepts related to the topic.

      7.   Now have the learners use a different color highlighter to mark the next most important fact/s and verbalize two or three sentences about it...then write it.
Alexander Graham Bell was born in Scotland in 1845. He visited his grandfather in England when he was fifteen. He was always interested in inventing things because his grandfather took him to an Inventor's Museum. When he came back from Scotland he tried to invent a machine with a voice, with his brothers' help.

      8.   Next have the learners use another color highlighter, mark the next most important fact/s, and verbalize again several sentences about it...then write it.
Bell's mother was deaf and his father was a teacher of deaf children. This is probably why he decided to become a teacher of the deaf. He went to the United States and worked as a teacher while he worked on his inventions at night.

      9. Ask the learner to use a fourth color to mark the last information that should be included in the writing.
Bell worked very hard with his inventions. He had a friend named Tom Watson who helped him. They finally got a patent for the telephone in 1876.

10.   Encourage the learners to make a final summary sentence that gives the lesson or impact of the topic. *We all appreciated Alexander Graham Bell because he made our lives better by making the first telephone.*

Using the W-Guide as a format for a composition, contributes to developing the understanding that writing is a process. Until the steps in the process become automatic, learners will need to use a strategy to be productive. When they have rehearsed the technique and use it easily, they can begin to skip steps in the process. Actually the steps will become intuitive and they will be unaware that they are actually using them any longer. For instance, instead of highlighting the items in the chart, they will automatically see what is important and work directly from the chart in grouping their thoughts and content. The process will become simpler and more efficient as they become experienced in using it.

TIME AND SPACE CONCEPTUALIZATION

Understanding where we are in both time and space is an attribute of being centered or grounded. Many of our learners, as they were sharing their frustrations, described the confusion they experienced in knowing where they were in space. They did not have a conceptualization of direction.. They did not know the direction of the grocery store from where they were. They could not point in the direction of another city. They were not oriented in space.

Others shared their confusion about time. They were unable to schedule their day, week, or lives. They did not understand how long it would take to complete a project or a task. They often found that it took much longer than they had estimated and they were overwhelmed with too much to do.

Time and space conceptualization is an essential attribute for us to possess for efficient and effective working and living skills. The interventions will appear obvious. They are effective in changing these skills.

Space Conceptualization

> *Ron - I drove away from here last week and got on the freeway to the left. I was certain that I was headed in the right direction but it began to feel strange because it didn't look familiar.*

> *JS - You were leaving Sacramento to go to San Francisco, is that correct?*

> *R - Yes, but it turns out I was headed toward Stockton. I eventually got turned back around but it made me mad.*

185

JS - You have shared before that direction was a hassle for you.

R - It has always been a mystery to me.

JS - Can you read a road map?

R - Not easily, but eventually I can make sense of it.

JS - Let's get out a map of northern California. Would you locate where you are now...

R - Yes, here is Sacramento.

JS - What direction is it to San Francisco?

R - Well, that is odd. I always thought it was directly west but it is actually a bit southwest of here.

JS - Good observation. Just for a moment, use your imagery and see yourself in relation to San Francisco. See where you are now. Image all that land in between until you come to San Francisco.

R - Yes, I see it.

186

JS - Now, image yourself driving out of the parking lot here. Which direction will you go?

R - First I turn left and then I go north on the freeway.

JS - Good. Now trace your path in the map in your head. See yourself making the turns even on the freeway. (Nodding) Stay oriented as though you were combining the map and the streets you see. Where are you now?

R - I can see the turn just as I come toward downtown. I have been going north, and now I am headed west.

JS - You can do this quite effectively. During the next week you will keep this at your level of conscious awareness, and think where you are in relation to a map or north/south orientation. You will know where you are all the time.

Establishing oneself in space requires an active awareness. It is only through this active effort that we can conceptualize space orientation. For younger or more involved learners, the orientation should begin at home. They should be able to draw their home. They should be able to stand facing a front door (or window or other wall) and image what is on the right, left, in front, or behind.   Once they can orient themselves within a confined space, they will need to orient themselves in relation to north, south, east and west. Quite often a city street map and a compass are helpful for this.

It is the dialoguing and active effort of orientation which is effective in developing this conceptualization. Developing a heightened sensitivity and provoking thinking, are both essential in creating orientation in space.

Time Conceptualization

Time understanding is a bit more complex for most learners. It requires two distinct concepts: an understanding of where we are in time and an understanding of how long different events or tasks require.

> *Tim - I am constantly scheduling myself to do several things at the same time. Everyone is often mad at me or I am rushing about trying to accomplish everything. Sometimes I buy tickets to a King's game, have a dinner party scheduled, and agree to a meeting all for the same evening. It is very frustrating to my family, and yet, I am just not aware of doing these things.*

Tim shared a perfect description of the confusion that occurs

188

for a learner when he does not remain conscious of time and where he is in time. Understanding time conceptualization requires both visual and language skills. We have to be able to *see* where we are in time or see the schedule for tomorrow or the next day. At the same time, we guide ourselves in moving through time with our language. We speak to ourselves and say...*at nine I have to be at the dentist, that will take about an hour; so by eleven I could be at the office to meet with the auditor; then I will have lunch at home at 12:30 and be back for the 1:30 meeting...etc.* Efficient processing allows us to *see* the schedule for the day and simultaneously talk about it.

<u>Daily Planning</u>

In order to plan a day, the integration of auditory and visual conceptualization is important. This is apparent in the dialogue with Tim regarding his schedule.

> *JS - Let's do some work with your time conceptualization. I notice you have a schedule book with you.*
>
> *T - Yes, I would be lost without it. I have to write everything down.*
>
> *JS - But you still over-schedule yourself?*

189

Learning Victories

    T - Well, yes, I forget to look at my schedule.

    JS - Ah, you are inconveniently normal! Let's look at your schedule today.. No, don't open your book. Just tell me about your schedule today as you know it.

    T - I started the day with a meeting at 8:00 and then I came here for 10:00 and I will go back to the bank; and there are meetings, but I am not sure when they are. I'd have to look.

    JS - How did you just recall your schedule..did you see it written out?

    T - No, I just kind of know what I did this morning but I am not sure about this afternoon.

    JS - May I look at the schedule for today with you? (Nods.) We are going to image it on my door. Let's segment the door into a hours of the day like a giant schedule, starting at 7:00 a.m. until 10:00 p.m. Can you do that? It looks like noon is just above the doorknob. Right?

    T - I think I have it.

    JS - Good.   Now put the pieces in the schedule that

190

you are certain about. Can you see the morning appointment written in? Now how about the next ones?

T - Okay, yes I see them.

JS - Would you get up and orient me, on the door, so I can see where we are in time?

T - Sure, up at the top I am getting up...breakfast by 7:15 and then I leave the house at 7:45 and I have a meeting at 8:00. My meeting lasts..I know, I left at about 9:30 to come here. Now when I leave here, yes, it is lunch right here. I will work in my office 'til about 4:00, then I have to be at a meeting at headquarters.

JS - Pause a moment. You see yourself working until 4:00 but you have to be at a meeting at 4:00 elsewhere. How is that working for you?

T - I'm usually late.... let's see I think it takes about twenty minutes to get there, so I will either get there at 4:20 or need to leave earlier!

JS - Could this be an issue in your time planning?

191

> *T - You mean do I plan for driving time. No, I usually don't. Everyone seems to be used to me arriving late. They rib me about it.*

> *JS - How would it feel to be on time?*

> *T - I would like it. I could relax a minute before the meeting starts. You know, get my papers organized.*

> *JS - What kind of image would it create?*

> *T - I guess my bosses would be impressed. They would know I was working on it.*

> *JS - Is it of value to you to do it? I ask because it will require some work and thinking on our part.*

> *T - Yes. I would like to feel in control of my time.*

> *JS - Okay, carry on with the schedule...*

There are several issues imbedded in Tim's lateness. One is a very real distractability which we discussed earlier. He is very impulsive and rapidly processes information. There is an emotional overlay related to his perception of himself and others' perceptions of him. There are people that rely on directing him and he might disappoint them if he becomes

192

self-reliant both at work and home. In a sense, he pleases them by being *needy of their direction.*

Our lives are filled with well-intentioned people who become enablers or supporters and allow us to continue with our inappropriate habits and skills. Once they are in place, it is very difficult for us to change, because we would have to disappoint these people ,by not being dependent upon them any longer. For this reason , it was important to ask Tim how serious he was in wanting to change the skill of time management. If he was getting attention that he liked from everyone reacting to his being late, he would not be inclined to change.

Once our learners have understood how to image their schedule for a day and talk through it, we ask them to begin every day by doing that. As soon as they wake in the morning, they are instructed to image their schedule for the day. They must review the visual image with language. The combination of the visual and auditory reinforcement is very powerful in instituting memory.

Weekly Schedule

The understanding of calendar and time is equally important for retaining a weekly sequence of events in one's memory. This does not mean that learners are asked to be able to recite

193

seven daily schedules. It does mean that they are aware of significant or important events during the week. These are usually events or activities which require pre-planning, preparation of materials, purchase of supplies or are significant to the learner.

For instance, if ten guests are invited for dinner on a Thursday, the week's schedule will include pre-planning activities. By Wednesday there will be shopping to do and a menu to plan. On Thursday, there may be baking in the morning and setting the table. The day will be scheduled, but there will also be activities on prior days, to be completed in preparation for the dinner party.

This is the type of planning Tim needed to use to prevent himself from double- or triple-scheduling an activity for an evening. He needs to keep a sense of the week's events current in his mind in order to prevent over-scheduling.

Exercises for this, usually relate to actual events in the learner's lives. However, a demonstration of the steps for retention can be provided and used for practice. An example is provided:

> *JS - Let's put some energy into recalling the important activities you have for this week. What will you be scheduling that you should keep in mind?*

194

T - I'm not sure what I have.

JS - Well, then I will provide you with some wonderful activities for this week. On Thursday, you will get to go to a play at the Civic Center and you have to be there at 7:30. Since it is a special event for you and your wife, you will want to take her to dinner. What time will you set the reservations for dinner and where?

T - Well, our favorite restaurant is downtown so we could just walk to the Civic Center. Probably we should eat around 6:15 and leave home at 5:45. That means I would have to leave work by 5:00 to change.

JS - That is Thursday but on Wednesday, you have a PTA meeting at school at 8:00 with your son. It is Open House and you are to bring a model of an airplane, because the children are studying aviation; and the teacher wanted a display, so your son volunteered. You don't have one at home so you will have to buy it and assemble it before the open house.

T - Sounds like my real life! Okay, I have to buy it this weekend and then have it together by Tuesday morning and take it and my son to school. Now I

> *have Sunday, Monday, Tuesday and Wednesday involved with that activity.*

> *JS - Can you see your week with these activities in place?*

> *T - I think so. I can see the Sunday schedule: going to the store with my son at 2:00 and then spending the afternoon putting the model together. On Monday evening, we will have to paint the model so I need to be home early and have dinner before 7:00 so he can help. Then Tuesday morning I have to get up earlier, so I can take him to school and go in with the model. Then I have Wednesday night at the open house, and then dinner and theater on Thursday. You know, I've not thought in this way before. It could really help me with my scheduling issues.*

These exercises provide our learners with a 0new focus on time. Learners enjoy gaining control over *time* in their lives and will continue to use the strategies.

In addition to learning to schedule and to organize time, learners need to have accurate conceptualizations about how long it takes to do something. It was first apparent with younger learners. They did not have any idea how long it took for something to happen or to do a task. When we asked them how long it took to sneeze or to hop on one foot, they often replied that it took minutes. They did not have accurate concepts regarding time. Not only was there confusion in conception of time but there was little ability to *sense* the amount of time that passed.

To develop the awareness and experience of time passing, a focus on this concept was established. There were two types of exercises that were important to do. The first is used to establish a sensory knowledge to predict the passing of time.

Predicting Time Passage

The first exercise requires the learner to start a stopwatch and turn away from it (or turn it over). When the learner thinks that one minute has passed, she turns back to check the watch and records the number of seconds on the clock. If the learner is consistently more than ten seconds off in estimating the time, the therapist needs to establish some strategies, for the learner to employ to estimate time.

Strategies to estimate the passing of time include: rhythmic counting by thousands while watching the clock, tapping in a rhythmic manner to the movement of the second hand on a clock, and/or walking (or rocking) in step to the movement of the second hand. Practice with these strategies assists in

197

creating awareness and experience, in understanding *seconds* and *minutes*.

In order to develop an understanding of longer periods of time such as an hour or several hours, the learner needs to establish relationships between known activities and the amount of time they take. For instance, the amount of time it takes for a half hour television show is often a time block to which a learner can relate. So is the amount of time it takes to sit down and eat lunch, to drive from home to a destination or to play a game of basketball. The activities should have a relevancy to the learner's experiences.

In order to formalize the instruction in time awareness, it is appropriate to provide the learner with a daily schedule sheet, and have him record the activities that he anticipates for the day (or for a period of the day). Then have him be very conscious of the clock all day, and record the actual times it took to do the activities that were suggested. When the learner is accurately predicting how long it will take to do tasks or activities, then the therapist may assume that an understanding is being developed for time awareness.

Calendar Knowledge

Many of our learners are confused about the passage of time indicated by days, weeks, and months. They do not have any idea how long it will be before a vacation, birthday or special event. They are unable to relate dates to the day of the week. Learners frequently tell us that the first of a month starts on a Monday. They are shocked when we do a calendar exercise with them, and they find that months start on different days of the week.

We use a clock face in the center of a large piece of paper as a form for a calendar. One o'clock begins with January, Two o'clock is February, etc. We put a paper with the following image just to the side of each numeral:

Month _____

Sun	Mon	Tues	Wed	Thurs	Fri	Sat

The learner looks at a current calendar and fills in the numerals for the days of the week. Although it would be simpler to provide the calendar sheets for the learner, he would not be gaining the experience of placement of the dates. As we come to holidays or other significant dates we prompt the learner to recognize them. For each month we ask if there are any holidays, family events or birthdays? We also ask for the learner to identify vacation periods. If the learner is a student, then the year has significant benchmarks with the start of a semester, breaks, finals, report card periods, etc. These should all be noted on the calendar so that they can be tracked.

In the same way that a learner experiences confusion with the calendar, he will have difficulty with the concept of *seasons.* Most learners associate seasons with weather. While this is related to the seasons, the calendar is actually a more accurate monitor. Once the time clock with the calendar is completed, it is appropriate to divide the clock into quadrants which are representative of the seasons. This provides a graphic visualization of the information, and is effective in establishing the concept in a concrete manner.

SUMMARY

Edu-therapeutics addresses these areas of intervention to improve the learner's skills in independent performance. By establishing the processing skills and strategies for learning, the learner gains control and becomes effective in employing learning strategies for success. Strategies for developing memory, attention, processing (executive-function skills), and academics, are included in *You Don't Have to Be Dyslexic.*

Chapter Nine

LEARNING VICTORIES

Victory comes to learners in small doses, in massive differences and with peace in place of fear. Each of our learners has enjoyed the prospect of change which occurs during the learning process. It is with great joy that we share the victories our learners have experienced.

Change is often more apparent to the observer than the participant. I frequently see frustrations and complaints subside to be replaced with higher level desires and goals. I have found that the *absence of confusion and fear* is often difficult to register. It is much like a physical pain; we have difficulty recalling once it is gone. We know that there was something and it was unpleasant, but the intensity and limitations it posed have faded, as has the memory. It is the good fortune of our learners to experience the fading of the frustration and fear.

When Tim began to function more effectively in his scheduling and processing, his attendance faded. His need for reinforcement and continuing assistance diminished. As a therapist, I rejoiced as this happened.

Dear Dr. Smith:

I suppose I needed to write to you because I'm more than a bit embarrassed that I haven't followed through on our program in the last several months. This embarrassment is especially uncomfortable because you have been so instrumental in my recent growth and have been so unconditionally giving. Further, I realize that you will be leaving me soon and I haven't even come close to sharing how much I appreciate all that you've done for me. While it is probably in your nature to give to others, I've trained myself not to expect such support, and now want to convey to you how touched I am for all that you've done.

As for my progress with my attention issues, I am quite pleased to say that a strong common thread has woven its way into my life. With the skills that I learned with you, combined with my antidepressant, it now strongly appears that the major elements of my awareness are connected. It is now natural for me to transition between the major categories of my life (administrative, career, social, recreational, etc.) without getting lost in the minutia. I <u>sense</u> these categories rather than having the constant struggle of trying to maintain my awareness of them. My life *performance has improved substantially...and just in time.*

I am 80% of the way through opening my own marketing business. While I've always had many projects going at one time, I have never marched so unwaveringly through the necessary tasks. There is still help needed in my more moment-to-moment attention span. While distractability has indeed improved, it is still present. As long as it takes, I will work to correct these remaining attention and esteem issues.

Tim has discovered the power of his organization. After years of wanting to establish his own business, he has taken the necessary steps. As he continues to learn about himself, he will discover his incredible power and brilliance. He is learning about himself, one step at a time. It is a process.

Confidence in learning and performing does not come quickly. It is established quietly and secretly. It often sneaks up on a learner long after its presence is desired. Mark experienced several major life changes in the midst of his programming. His position was eliminated in a corporate downsizing, his wife was transferred to another state, and he became responsible for his father's care. He was challenged to use his extensive resources for coping with change. He was effective in facing these changes. His incredible spirit, talent, and soul emerged in a birthday card he prepared for me.

> *The Birthday Alchemist*
> *Turns time into gold*
> *Days become discoveries,*
> *Weeks become wonders,*
> *Months become magic,*
> *And years*
> *turn round and round*
> *in a dance*
> *with the soul of the world.*

So many of the learners who experience differences in their learning are blessed with creative and artistic attributes. It is possibly this difference which sensitizes them to the demands of the world. Whether they have strengths in creating with words, pictures, or ideas, they are wonderfully bright. As they realize their power as learners, they develop a depth in all of their attributes which was previously unrecognized.

Melody, a teacher and writer, confronted me on her fourth session, with a paper which had words crossed out all over it. Her frustration and anger oozed from every part of her body; her eyes, her lips, her posture. *Look at this. Just look at this. It's all scribbles. I can't get a coherent thought together!*

She was attempting to write about her trip to Yosemite. She greatly admired the writings of John Muir and was inspired to record her passionate feelings about the beauty of her surroundings. When she could not do that even in the peaceful environment she treasured, she reacted with great frustration and anger.

It was important for Melody to realize that her frustration was related to the slow response time which she experienced. She was unable to retrieve and process information efficiently. As Melody experienced changes in her processing through diet control and a new understanding of her talents, her writing changed. Later, she shared, *When I stop fighting myself, it does come out. I have had a few erasures, but it was not with any sense of panic or any sense of being critical about it.* And it did emerge as follows:

Meadow Musing

I am very glad to have found this meadow away from the noisy buses and endless stream of cars. It is no small miracle that none of the other fifteen thousand people here have discovered this patch of heaven. So I am most grateful that the only sound that fills me up now, is the blessed voice of the wind making her kind and gentle way between the leaves of the trees beside me. In her passing she creates soft soul-soothing

206

lyrics that echo down deep in my heart. You are home, Melody.

The strong arms of the meadow have gathered me in and wrapped me up in the past. A great mass of towering stones with waterfalls plunging down their granite walls, encompass me about like an army of watchful Angels. Their voices blend with the wind song to carry each of my worries far away. Even the sun is singing along, for the clouds have been chased away *and the river is dancing with the diamonds of light that the sun so freely gives. "Rise up our dear friend," the song seems to say, "and rejoice in our beauty which the Lord has made." And so I rise and run to the center of the meadow and stop still. What can mere mortal words say to describe such a holy moment. Silence would be a more honorable response. Yet knowing the limit of the words that are to follow, I feel impelled to go on. In that moment I could not speak or move, for great showers streamed down upon me to every pore and cell of my need, until my heart was near to bursting. All the wonders of the meadow had come together to infuse me with their gifts of joy and light, comfort and strength, wisdom and healing. Divine touching mortal, making us one. Can there be any other moment as sacred?*

> *I long for more of such moments in my life. I think*
> *they are more available to us than we can wildly*
> *imagine, and I think that we do not even have to have*
> *a meadow, for I believe that this stream pours down*
> *upon us all without end. There are but two things*
> *required of us; to open our hearts to the stream, be*
> *still, and listen. If we can do both of these things long*
> *enough, our holy moments will come in many*
> *surprising ways, because quite unlike words, they*
> *have no limits.*

The powerful confidence Melody exhibited in her writing,
reflected the strength that was within her. It is in such
contrast to her observations of herself prior to learning about
her attributes.

> *I started to become increasingly aware and frustrated*
> *with how I learn a few years ago when I considered*
> *going to grad school. I realized that because I had*
> *to read material over and over again to understand*
> *it, that I needed a more efficient way to take in*
> *information. I also began to become more aware of*
> *long-standing difficulties, in other areas. For as far*
> *back as I could remember, I had felt frustrated*
> *because I couldn't comprehend information I received*
> *verbally or through reading "fast enough." I also*
> *had difficulty remembering what I heard or read, even*

immediately afterwards. It took me long periods of time to formulate and organize my thoughts, when I wanted to express my thinking, either in verbal or written form. I felt as if the information was all floating around, and I was unable to grab on to the pieces to put them together into a whole, or to determine the important information from the unimportant. I thought that there was something wrong with me and that in reality I was stupid.

I also realized that at work I was very frustrated with the amount of time it took me to problem-solve, evaluate, and analyze information. As a teacher, I wanted these skills. I rarely offered suggestions or opinions at staff meetings because I could not trust my judgements. I had difficulty attending to the spoken word, not only in work situations, but in casual conversations. I would catch the beginnings and ends, but within one to three minutes, lose the middle part of what was being said. My coping strategy, so that people would not know that I lost them, was to repeat the last two or three things that they said. Perhaps this was part of the reason I became a quiet person. I didn't know what had been said, so I wasn't sure how to respond. When I did take the chance to say something, many times I felt I

> *had said something stupid and would go home and cry at night over my errors. I often heard, "Why don't you think before you talk?"*

Many learners will listen to Melody's story and recognize the pain and frustration as their own. As a learner, Melody could only elaborate on her needs because they appeared to overshadow her talents and skills. She was unaware of the full range of her attributes. When she began to recognize that she possessed a full-range of attributes, her focus shifted.

> *By the time I came to Melvin-Smith, I knew that I wanted to make some changes, but had almost given up hope that it was possible to think or learn in significantly different ways. What a tremendous relief to find, on my first day, that there were actual, valid reasons for all my frustrations and that something could be done to change them. It had been a long search. I still had reasonable doubts.*

> *From the first, every exercise we did was empowering. They were concrete contradictions to what I believed about my thinking. The visual memory cards, with and without words, gave me immediate, indisputable feedback that my memory could work well. Shifting the pictures around was a vivid lesson in flexible thinking, showing me*

> *possibilities beyond the linear way of thinking that I had felt most comfortable with.*

As therapists, we cannot tell a learner that they are smart or that they can do something. They must experience it themselves. They must discover that they can be successful and effective. They must convince themselves in order to recognize that they are effective learners.

> *The learning and insights gained from the Mind Benders was astonishing to me. I realized the second day of working with them that they caused me to panic. It was a quiet panic. One that I had grown accustomed to feeling without even being aware of it. And I didn't want anyone to know that I didn't feel capable or smart enough to do these things. I thought about catching the next plane back home. There weren't any of these "things" there. These would require me to work on my thinking function, because there was no way my emotion could be of any help whatsoever.*

> *My breathing became shallow, my thinking shut down. And I wasn't even aware of either of those things happening until we discussed it, Joan. And then I realized that this was my automatic response to the majority of situations that required me to use*

211

> *logical reasoning. So the first thing you taught me to do was breathe... to keep the thinking process going and to give myself time.*

Shallow breathing reduces the oxygen that is being delivered to the brain. It inhibits the effective activation of brain cells by reducing their ability to be energized. It is a common reaction to fear and frustration. Since it reduces thinking function, it inhibits performance. Thus the learner feels justified in the fear of failure and begins to generalize it to all activities of this type.

> *One of the first strategies you and John taught me was to experiment, to help myself discover the answer. This was a totally new concept to me, as a valid way to solve a problem. I thought I had to get the answer right the first time, which you soon helped me to discover was perfectionism.*

> *Experimenting allowed for the freedom to explore, to try out different solutions without fear of mistakes, to be flexible and "play" with the information. Play? Have fun? Not me. Thinking was hard work. Hadn't I proved that for the last, oh, thirty years or so? Well, maybe it could be fun...perfectionism certainly wasn't a laugh-a-minute and I had always been afraid of making mistakes.*

We have done a true disservice to our learners by teaching them that there is a *right answer*, that there is *only one* right answer. Certainly, this type of teaching limits exploration and creates fear in learners of *being wrong*. We need to teach our learners that there are many answers, and to choose the most appropriate answer sometimes requires exploration.

> *I learned that I could not solve the puzzles with one swift answer. I was forced to accept the fact that it would take time to work through them, and this allowed me to give myself permission to process, which I had not been able to do before. I immediately saw how I could start applying these strategies to everyday life. I never dreamed that these things would hold so many treasures!*

> *There was another important something happening. You had shared the results of your research about the effects of diet on the thinking processes. I made the decision to omit dairy products and sugar from my diet. It would be an experiment. I didn't really expect to find any significant difference in the way I felt or how I processed information.*

> *You gave me the TOVA on the first day, and we were to repeat it on the last day of our programming two weeks later. I was in for a surprise and my slight*

213

skepticism was cured. When I looked at the differences, I could hardly believe my eyes. My processing time had gone down by almost double.

Writing this after continuing to remain dairy and sugar-free for seven weeks, I have more energy now than I have ever felt. At work, I would experience a big "down time" after lunch on a daily basis. That no longer happens. I have noticed a definite difference in my processing time, and have been able to problem-solve, analyze and evaluate more quickly and efficiently.

Two days after I returned from California, I gave an overview of the work we had done, and then gave an hour and a half in-depth presentation the following day on specific exercises we had done. I did both with little preparation and felt very organized, comfortable and confident each time. I must say, it flowed very nicely. But, speaking to a group of adults is something I had successfully avoided since college. When required to do the dreaded task, I would spend weeks preparing and worrying about it. So, Joan, you can imagine how I felt when I was able to do this without any anxiety at all.

Adjusting diet, and eliminating two of the most rewarding and pleasing items from the diet, is incredibly difficult. It would probably be much easier for most people to give up vegetables or salads or any other food group than *sugar!* Even though we can prove the differences in response time and performance when a learner monitors his or her diet, it is very difficult to sustain. Our society has an incredible addiction to sugar. We consume considerable amounts of it at every meal. It is only when we begin looking at the information labels on products that we realize how much we consume.

> *I feel that as a direct result of the interventions at Melvin-Smith, I have more confidence in my thinking abilities than I could have ever hoped to achieve. I now know that I think well, so my old , negative message no longer has any power over me. It has been healed. I don't have to look outside myself anymore to get approval of how I think. The gap between my feeling and thinking functions is closing. I have learned to respect my emotional center for the valuable feedback it can give me. I know that it will continue to play an important role in my decisions. But before, using that center was my only option, leaving me without choices. And where there are no choices, there is fear. Joan, I'm not afraid anymore.*

215

Learning Victories

There is a common theme of *fear* that each of our learners has shared. What a dramatic emotion to be associated with a simple inefficiency in an attribute. The real impact of this subtle difference in learning is immense. It is powerful and debilitating.

Liz completed her programming and decided to become a specialist in remediation of dyslexia. She found that she had many talents to share, and the confidence to experiment with teaching emerged for her. Her words relay the tremendous changes she has experienced.

> *This letter is about my transformation; and about still-water ripples that spread from a single pebble; and about doing unto others; and about what goes around comes around; and about passing good on, hand-to-hand, one at a time.*
>
> *My first memory is from inside the buggy: a flash of awareness, a visual image of the hood above my eyes and the side metal supports. I may have changed the "address" of this memory over the years, updated its location with the development of my intellect, ` but the picture is whole, real and still has the emotional power of that brilliant moment of waking. It was the herald for a skill I misplaced for a long time. A skill I set aside, to work very hard at processing*

216

information the way I thought other people did. With your support and training, I have found the skill again, along with so much more.

Liz recognized that her attributes and talents in visualization had been long denied. She attempted to learn through her auditory system - a system which was not particularly powerful for her. She was meant to be a visual learner.

Growing up, I had worked very hard to make it easy for myself. I worked very hard because I knew, on some level of awareness, the truth in messages like "she could be doing much better" and "she is actually very bright." The labels were the toughest..."lazy" and "underachiever", for example. I learned to compensate; developed a complex system to add and subtract numbers when flash cards didn't help; to read paragraphs over and over to make sure I wasn't missing a key point. I learned when to nod to buy processing time in conversations when I actually didn't have a clue. The compensations were sometimes effective and sometimes disastrous (sometimes I was "found out"). However, thinking about changing them was like leaping from a cliff.

I look back at how it felt to take the first step, to take the risk, to take the test. Contemplating objective

217

> *validation for the "lazy" label was daunting. "What if the test showed there was nothing wrong?" This angst, even though I knew, somewhere deep, that I was definitely not lazy. I had to work very hard at some things to even keep up, and there were things, like Blackjack, I avoided altogether to protect me from embarrassment.*

How different our lives are when we experience fear and embarrassment. When we are constantly on-guard to keep from making a mistake, we experience continual stress. It is unnecessary for any learner to have to live with such tension when we understand how to relieve these symptoms.

> *Now, after our work together, I have changed and continue to change. I used to assume I was the one who hadn't gotten it "right", who didn't understand. I am gaining more and more confidence. Sometimes, actually often, I did get it, I did understand. There were actually very good reasons for me to draw the conclusions or do what I did. I am beginning to value and explain my rationale. Now I know about "evidence"...about, trusting my evidence. This has wide-ranging implications. I used to look for something in the same pile of papers, over and over and over, used to circle the block, over and over and over, following directions that weren't working. I*

218

used to fill in the things I didn't understand in a conversation, sometimes incorrectly and to my embarrassment.

Analyzing evidence includes the ability to examine a process I am using and evaluate its effectiveness. Then, if it's not working, switch processes...change approaches. Part of this is sticking with a process longer, and being able to evaluate what is and is not working, and make the adjustment accordingly.

Now I also realize that sometimes people without the same imaginative, visual approach to information have difficulty "tracking" with me. I can take information, current facts and project into the future, given those facts. The results - I make leaps in logic that are actually correct, and sometimes it takes others awhile to fill in the blanks I've been able to visualize. Sometimes just describing the pictures, describing what I see as I "run the movie", beginning to end, leads to understanding.

Liz possesses a powerful ability to visualize information. She is now using it for her benefit instead of denying it and attempting to suppress it. It has given her a new power in performing effectively at work, home and in her mentoring program.

219

After our work together, I'm doing things I would not have attempted before. I've joined Toastmasters and prepare speeches or speak spontaneously. Both require taking the pictures from my head and changing them to words in a way others can understand. It's the "language piece" that is so much more than simply learning to talk. I am a student hot air balloon pilot. I was able to take 24 hours of ground school in two days, and learn to retain enough highly technical information about reading aviation weather reports, flight instruments, etc., to pass the Federal Aviation Administration pilot test.

I used skills honed by our work to lay a ceramic tile floor in my bathroom. I "ran the movie", pictured the steps in order, beginning to end, (it was the plan) to identify all the equipment and supplies, and to predict and prepare for likely problems. Memorization by pictures is a magical skill for me. Now I remember things and give directions straight from images rather than feeling panicky about coming up with the "right" words.

A very helpful result is my growing ability to separate when my dyslexic learning style has "kicked in", and when others are not communicating in a way I can understand. Social situations are still a little befuddling. People talk fast, they talk in code, and sometimes I don't "catch it" (sometimes others don't either) but at least I know what is happening and that makes it easier. There are also things I do catch.

Listening to Liz's confidence and understanding assists us in appreciating the changes which she has experienced. She recognizes that perfection is not an ideal. She expects no more of herself than of others. She realizes the fragility of skills and embraces this wonderful imperfection in others, too.

Now I am a mentor, "buddy", to Adam, a first grader who knows a lot about things...King Neptune, armadillos and sharks, and skipping rocks... but very little about reading and counting. We need each other. In six months, he has gone from barely speaking and acting out his frustrations as his very capable brain leaps, faster than I can shift, from one very interesting thing to the next. I am learning understanding and patience, and a certain amount of humility. I am everlastingly amazed at the way core intellect and the human spirit survive. I've committed to hanging in there with him; to offering up my experience to help him learn; to letting him take from me what he can use; to helping him accept the wonderful and unique individual he is. The pebble

221

is dropped. The ripples have begun.

This is a thank you letter; a thank you letter for whatever awareness and understanding I can pass to others. Most especially, however, this is a thank you letter for my freedom.

I believe that learning is the power to freedom. I believe that we all have the potential and the control within our grasp to be unique and successful learners. I believe that, for me, it is necessary to share how to make this happen, so that we can inspire new believers. They, in turn, will reach new learners and set them free to learn.

Bibliography and Recommended Reading

Ayres, Jean. *Sensory Integration and Learning Disorders.* Los Angeles, CA: Western Psychological services, 1975.

Conners, C. Keith. *Feeding the Brain.* New York: Plenum Press, 1989.

Critical Thinking Books and Software Catalogue. 495 Elder Avenue, Sand City, CA., 831-393-3288. (Mind Benders).

Crook, Wm. G. *Help for the Hyperactive Child.* Jackson, Tenn: Professional Books, 1991.

Davis, Ronald. *The Gift of Dyslexia.* San Juan Capistrano, CA: Ability Workshop Press, 1994.

Duffy, Frank and Geschwind, Norman. *Dyslexia: A Neuroscientific Approcah to Clinical Evaluation.* Boston: Little, Brown and Co., 1985.

Ekstein, Rudolf. *Children of Time, space, Action, and Impulse.* New York: Appleton Centruy Crofts, 1966.

Greenberg, Lawrence. *Test of Variables of Attention, TOVA. Los Alamitis, CA., Unviersal Attention Disorders, 1996.*

Hamilton, Kirk. *The Experts Speak: The Role of Nutrition in*

Medicine. Sacramento, CA.: IT Services, 1996.

Healy, Jane. *Endangered Minds.* New York: A Touch Stone Book, Simon and Schuster, 1990.

Healy, Jane. *Your Child's Growing Mind.* New York: Doubleday and Co., 1987.

Hersey, Jane. *Why Can't My Child Behave.* Alexandria, VA: Pear Tree, 1996.

Hills, Sandra and Wyman, Pat. *Whats Food Got To Do With It?.* Windsor, CA: Center for New Discoveries in Learning, 1997.

Levine, Mel. *Keeping Ahead in School.* Cambridge, MA: Educational Publishing Services, Inc., 1990.

Levinson, Harold N. *Total Concentration.* New York: M. Evans and Company, 1990.

Luvmour, Josette and Luvmour, Sambhava. *Natural Learning Rhythms.* Berkeley, CA.: Celestial Arts, 1993

Lyon, G. Reid. *Attention, Memory and Executive Function.* Baltimore, Maryland: Paul H. Brookes Publishing Co., 1996.

Rochlitz, Steven. *Allergies and Candida*. New York: Human Ecology Balancing Sciences Inc., 1995.

Rapp, Doris. *Is This Your Child*. New York: Wm. Morrow, 1991.

Rosenthal, Joseph H. *The Neuropsychopathology of Written Language*. Berkeley: Rosenthal, 1977.

Shea, Charles, Shebilske, Wayne, and Worchel, Stephen. *Motor Learning and Control*. New Jersey: Prentice Hall, 1993.

Silver, Larry B. *Attention-Deficit Hyperactive Disorder*. Washington, D.C.: American Psychiatric Press, 1992.

Smith, Joan M. *Competency Assessment Battery - Computerized Program for Diagnostic Training*. Sacramento, CA.: Learning Time Products, Inc. 1997.

Smith, Joan M. *Easing Into Reading - Developing Beginning Skills Manual and Materials*. Sacramento, CA: Learning Time Products, Inc. 1996.

Smith, Joan M. *Memory Training Manual*. Sacramento, CA: Learning Time Products, Inc. 1996.

Smith, Joan M. *The Auditory Phonics Program - Reading Manual.* Sacramento, CA: Learning Time Products, Inc. 1994.

Smith, Joan M. *You Don't Have To Be Dyslexic.* Sacramento, CA.: Learning Time Products, Inc. 1993.

Tallal, Paula. *Fast ForWord.* Reference: Scientific Learning Corporation, Berkeley, CA. 1998. http://www.fastforword.com/

Content Guide

About Melvin-Smith Learning Centers
Creating Brighter Futures

The Melvin-Smith Learning Centers were established in 1968 to provide diagnosis, intervention, research, and materials to resolve inefficiencies associated with learning disabilities, dyslexia and attention-hyperactive disorders. The centers are operated by Learning Time, a California Nonprofit, tax-exempt organization.

The Centers have served over 15,000 learners during the past thirty years. They provide services directly in clinic, private parochial, and public school settings. The clinics provide one-to-one training programs and offer intensive services for learners from outside the geographical areas where clinics are located.

Learning Time provides professional training for teachers and parents to remediate learning inefficiencies. Edu-Therapeutics is taught in the training programs and a certificate program is offered as described on the next page.

Edu-Therapeutics materials are available through the centers. The Competency Assessment Battery provides a computerized program for evaluation of learner attributes. Companion materials and Training Cards enable professionals and parents to implement Edu-Therapeutic techniques for student success.

230

Where to Learn **Edu-Therapeutics**

Edu-Therapeutics is the content for the ***Dyslexia Remediation Specialist Certificate Program***. The program provides five courses which prepare teachers, therapists, psychologists and parents to use the techniques from Edu-Therapeutics. The training addresses dyslexic, attention deficit disorder and other learning challenges which are commonly identified as *learning disabilities.* Specialists learn to identify the attributes which are required for learning, evaluate processing inefficiencies, and implement programs to develop memory, attention, executive function skills, and unique reading spelling, writing and math systems to increase learning. Courses are presented in seven day intensive series in Sacramento and Monterey, California.

"This training gave me a whole new bag, filled with precise instruments for instruction. It cuts to the core percepts of learning..the processing of language and improvement of memory and attention skills. With it comes a fresh new outlook toward how learning happens. I can now achieve my goal of having my children emerge from the educational experiences with their self-esteem and excitement intact!"

Resource Specialist Teacher

Learner Intensives

The Melvin-Smith Learning Centers provide Intensive Programs for learners who are anxious to rapidly develop their learning skills or who are at a distance from a center or therapist. The training program requires a three to five week commitment of three hours daily (M-F) in Sacramento or Monterey. Intensive programs are designed to identify the learner's attributes and provide programming to resolve areas of inefficiency.

The learner will need to engage in on-going development work at the conclusion of the intensive to assure comfortable access to learning skills and develop automatic response levels. During the last week of training a person who can coach the learner, such as: a parent, teacher, or volunteer, should accompany the learner to receive training to implement on-going interventions.

Learner's with multiple issues often use the Intensive period for diagnostic learning. During this process, specialists evaluate the learner's skills and design and implement a program to increase efficiency. A teacher or specialist participates with the learner in order to be able to implement the program .

For Information: 1-800-50-LEARN
http://www.edu-therapeutics.com

232

CENTRAL